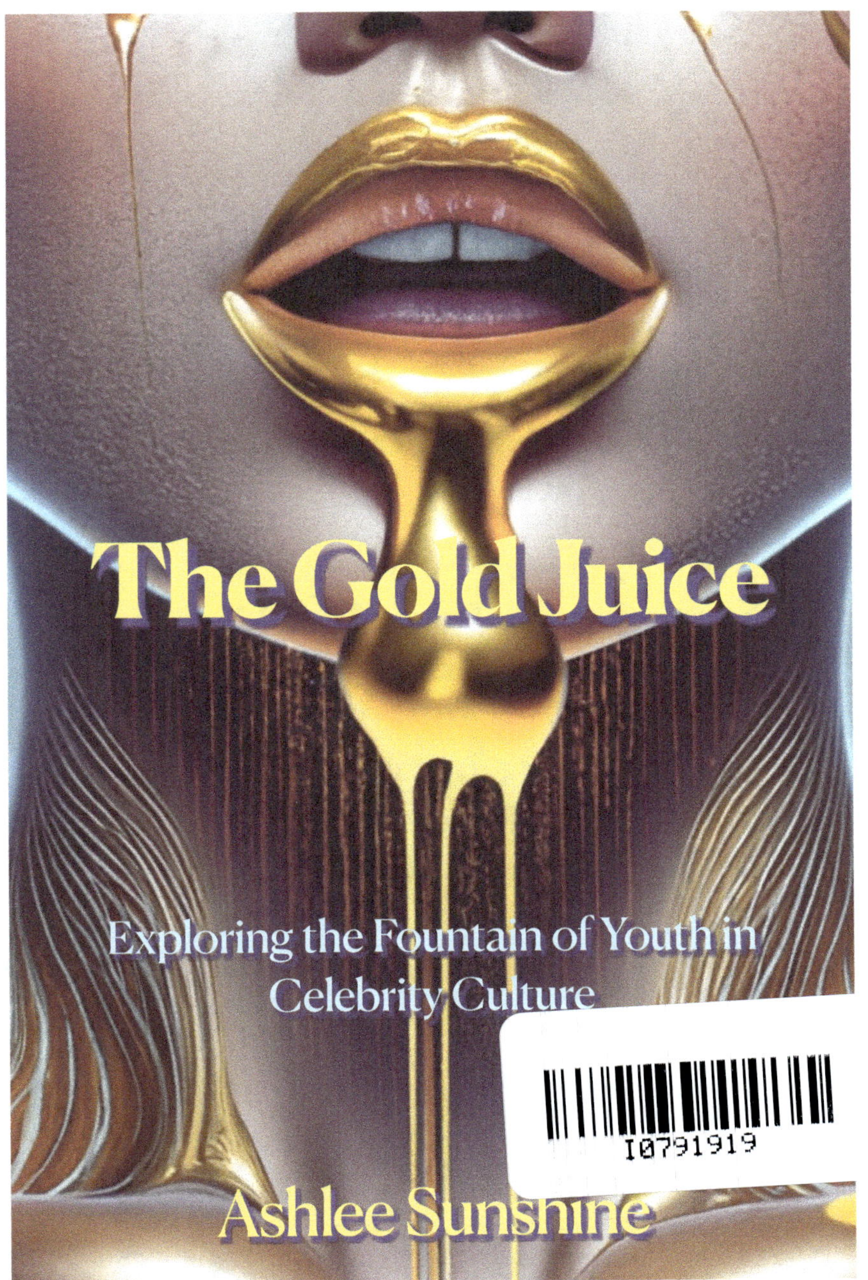

The Gold Juice
Exploring the Fountain of Youth in Celebrity Culture
Ashlee Sunshine

Ashlee Sunshine

The Gold Juice

Ashlee, the visionary behind Sunshine Paradise Retreat and an experienced Holistic Lifestyle Guide based in the vibrant city of Los Angeles, California, brings a unique blend of expertise and a worldly perspective to her work. Driven by a deep passion for guiding others toward peace, balance, and well-being, Ashlee has dedicated her life to helping individuals reconnect with themselves and the world around them. This book is both an educational and entertaining exploration of human nature and society's enduring fascination with immortality, offering insights and inspiration for anyone on the path of self-discovery and growth.

Ashlee Sunshine
www.sunshineparadiseretreat.com

Table of Contents

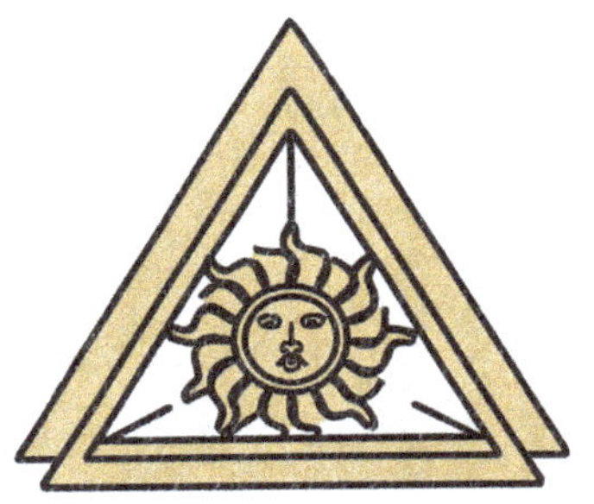

"There is a Fountain of Youth:
It is your mind, your talents, the creativity you
bring to your life and the lives of people you
love. When you learn to tap this source, you will
truly have defeated age."
-Sophia Loren

Introduction

Taryn Manning: "You don't drink the Kool-Aid; you don't drink the gold juice. So, I was offered the gold juice three times in my 20s, my 30s, and my 40s."

Whitney Cummings: "What's that? Pee? Lot of golden showers."

Taryn Manning: "The gold juice. That I will live forever and I'll have whatever I want. The gold juice. You never got offered the gold juice?"

Whitney Cummings: "No! I'm a scumbag comic. What's the gold juice?"

Taryn Manning: "Mmmm, I don't know, I don't know, but I didn't drink it and I didn't want it, and I noticed when all the girls, certain girls on Orange, changed. Yeah, this is a real thing, it's like a real thing, like it's all a real thing and it's scary because they send like people after you and they can kind of moonlight as like a friend or, you know, and they're a wolf in sheep's clothing and listen you can have everything you want, all the fame in the world, all the money. I'm like hmmm... what if I just drank it, but then you know what I mean? Like what if I and I don't know what it is. If it's a metaphor for the gold juice like you feel what I'm saying?"

Whitney Cummings: "If there's a tincture that makes you younger, I better know where you better let me in on this. If adrenochrome is real, let me in on this."

The above conversation is between Taryn Manning and Whitney Cummings on Whitney's podcast.

It was November 2023 when I first stumbled across a clip of Taryn Manning on Whitney Cummings' podcast that had taken TikTok by storm. In the video, she was raving about something called "gold juice." The clip was only about 15 seconds long, but it was enough to spark my curiosity—and apparently, I wasn't the only one. Everyone in the comments seemed equally intrigued, throwing around guesses and theories about what this mysterious drink could be. I had never heard of "gold juice" before, but the more these clips showed up on my feed, the more I felt drawn to dig deeper and figure out what all the fuss was about.

I dove headfirst into an internet deep dive, determined to figure out what was really going on with this strange phenomenon. The more I searched, the more fascinating—and honestly, bizarre—things I found. It felt like I had opened a door to a whole other world of theories, stories, and explanations. I should mention, though, that not everything I came across seemed entirely credible. Mixed in with the more grounded ideas were some truly wild conspiracy theories—don't worry, I'll unpack those later in the book. For now, let's just say the journey to uncover the truth behind "gold juice" turned out to be far more intriguing than I expected.

After diving into all my research, I felt like I had to share what I'd learned. So, I wrote a blog post about the "gold juice" phenomenon and published it on my yoga retreat website, SunshineParadiseRetreat.com. I broke everything down, from what sparked my curiosity to the wild theories I'd uncovered. To my surprise, the post blew up! By the time I sat down to write this book in April 2024, it had racked up an incredible 62,087 views. I never expected that kind of response, but it was clear this topic had captured a lot of people's attention—just like it had mine.

As an artist, I couldn't help but feel inspired by the idea of "gold juice." It sparked my creativity, leading me to design a series of artistic images that tried to capture its essence. I included these visuals in my blog post, hoping to add a unique, visual layer to my exploration of the topic. Imagine my excitement when I found out that Whitney Cummings had used one of my "gold juice" artworks as the cover photo for a follow-up podcast episode with Taryn Manning on her YouTube channel.

It felt surreal to see my work featured in such a big way! By the way, every image you see in this book is created by me—straight from my imagination to the page.

As I sit down to write this book, I want to invite you to come along with me on this journey. Together, we'll dive into the fascinating world of "gold juice," peeling back the layers of mystery and uncovering what makes this substance so intriguing. Along the way, we'll explore wild conspiracy theories, endless speculation, and humanity's timeless obsession with the quest for eternal youth. Through stories, ideas, and even a bit of art, we'll uncover what lies at the heart of this phenomenon. So, let's not waste any time—let's jump right in and discover the truth behind "gold juice.

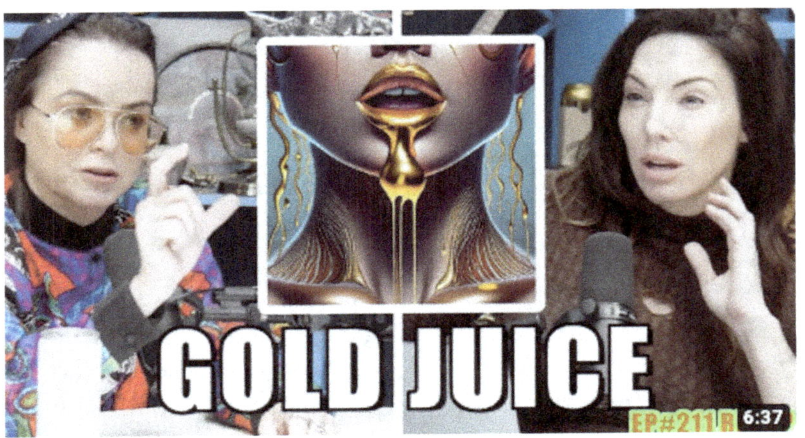

My gold juice image featured on the cover photo of Whitney Cummings Podcast episode on Youtube.

The Gold Juice Conspiracy Explained with Taryn Manning |

11K views • 1 month ago

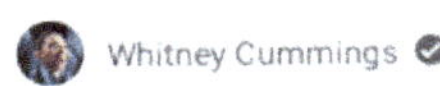 Whitney Cummings ✔

Guest star **Taryn Manning** opens up with Whitney Cummings about **the Gold Juice** conspiracy that is going on in Hollywood.

Chapter 1: Extreme Measures and Celebrity Secrets

Youth isn't defined by age; it's a mindset and a way of living.

Staying young isn't just a goal—it's an obsession for the rich and famous. From Hollywood stars to powerful influencers, those at the top will do just about anything to turn back the clock. They shell out big bucks on the latest anti-aging treatments, secret wellness retreats, and even dive into some pretty wild conspiracy theories. As we explore the depths of celebrity culture, we'll uncover the extreme steps and hidden secrets the rich and famous use to keep that youthful glow.

The Perilous Pursuit of Perfection

For the rich and famous, staying young is like hitting the jackpot. There's a side to this scene that's full of whispers and hidden truths. It's the world of extreme plastic surgeries, where stars and the elite are willing to go under the knife to try and stop time in its tracks.

Picture stepping into an operating room where the quest for eternal youth gets pretty intense. Here, the rich and famous trust top surgeons to help them chase perfection through a range of procedures. Facelifts, liposuction, nose jobs, breast enhancements—each surgery is a roll of the dice in their relentless pursuit to look flawless.

It's the over-the-top stories that really grab our attention. Rumors swirl about celebrities undergoing marathon surgery sessions, piling on multiple procedures at once in a desperate attempt to regain their youth. The operating room becomes their go-to place, and the surgeon acts like their trusted advisor as they take extreme measures chasing an unreachable ideal.

But it's not just how many surgeries they have—it's the types that make us do a double-take. Stories emerge of unusual procedures where implants seem to defy gravity and body proportions get seriously out of whack. Breasts enlarged to exaggerated sizes, noses reduced to tiny slivers, and faces turning into emotionless masks.

In this intense world where beauty and vanity mix, the line between improving and harming oneself starts to blur. The chase for perfection can turn into a shocking display, taking a heavy toll on both body and mind.

Hidden behind the facade of beauty, there's a darker truth—a story of pain, struggle, and an endless need for validation. In the world of extreme plastic surgeries, perfection comes at a cost paid not just in dollars, but in flesh and blood. As the quest for eternal youth continues, we can't help but wonder: what are we really sacrificing to chase this elusive dream of perfection?

Metamorphosis: The Dramatic World of Extreme Celebrity Makeovers

At first glance, Hollywood seems like a glamorous place, but when you look closer, you'll find a fascinating world of extreme makeovers and jaw-dropping surgeries. Celebrities often spare no expense to sculpt their bodies and faces, pushing cosmetic enhancements to the limit.

One of the most notable examples of a celebrity known for multiple plastic surgery transformations in a single session is the late pop icon Michael Jackson. Throughout his career, Jackson underwent several cosmetic procedures, including rhinoplasty (nose jobs), chin reshaping, and facial restructuring.

However, his most significant transformation occurred during the 1980s when he reportedly underwent extensive facial surgeries, including cheekbone implants, jawline reshaping, and skin bleaching. These dramatic changes to his appearance sparked widespread speculation and controversy, with many attributing his altered features to a combination of plastic surgery and skin condition. Despite the controversy, Jackson remained one of the most iconic figures in music history, leaving behind a complex legacy that continues to fascinate and intrigue fans worldwide.

Another prominent example is reality TV star and socialite, Heidi Montag. In 2010, Montag made headlines when she underwent a staggering ten plastic surgery procedures in a single day. These procedures included a mini brow lift, botox injections, nose job revision, chin reduction, ear pinning, breast augmentation revision, liposuction on her neck, waist, and thighs, as well as buttock augmentation. Montag's decision to undergo such extensive surgery sparked intense media scrutiny and raised questions about the potential risks and psychological motivations behind her drastic transformation. Despite facing criticism and health complications post-surgery, Montag has since spoken out about her experiences and the pressures she felt to conform to unrealistic beauty standards in Hollywood.

Valeria Lukyanova, frequently referred to as the "Human Barbie," stands out as another infamous example of extreme plastic surgery aimed at emulating a fictional character. Lukyanova gained international attention for her striking resemblance to the popular Barbie doll, achieved through a series of drastic cosmetic procedures that reportedly cost over a half-million dollars. From breast implants and rhinoplasty to waist reduction surgeries and extensive makeup, Lukyanova transformed herself into a living embodiment of the iconic toy. Her doll-like features, including large eyes, a tiny waist, and exaggerated proportions, captivated the public imagination, sparking debates about beauty standards and the lengths some individuals are willing to go to achieve them. While Lukyanova claims her body (besides her breasts) is all natural and a direct result of gym workouts and a particular diet, many are suspicious of her claims. Despite the controversy surrounding her transformation, Lukyanova's Barbie persona continues to fascinate and intrigue people around the world.

These examples highlight the extreme lengths to which some celebrities have gone in pursuit of physical perfection, often undergoing multiple plastic surgery procedures in a single session. While such transformations may temporarily alter their appearance, they also raise important questions about the societal pressures, psychological impact, potential risks associated with cosmetic enhancements in the entertainment industry.

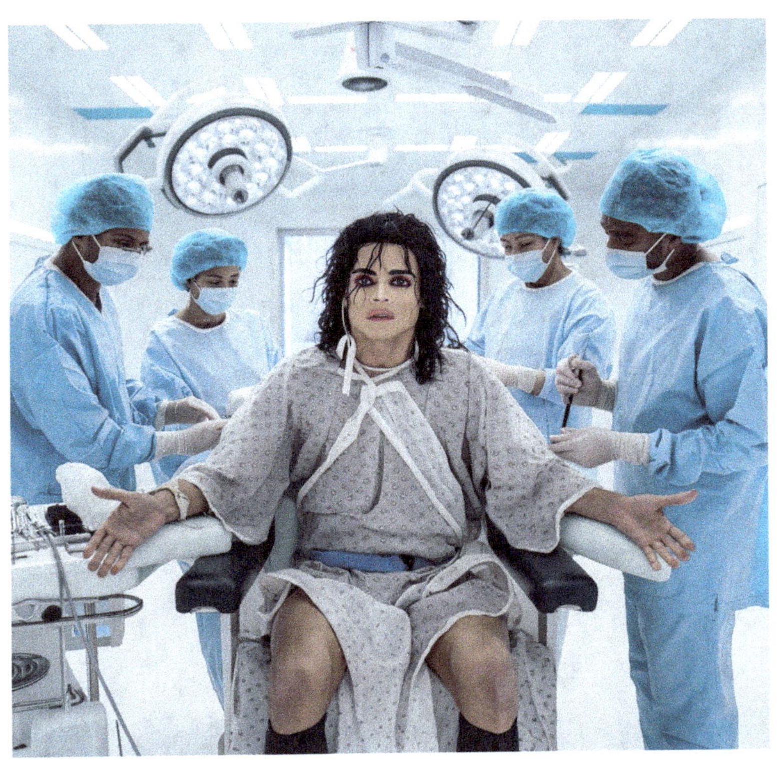

Shaping Michael Jackson

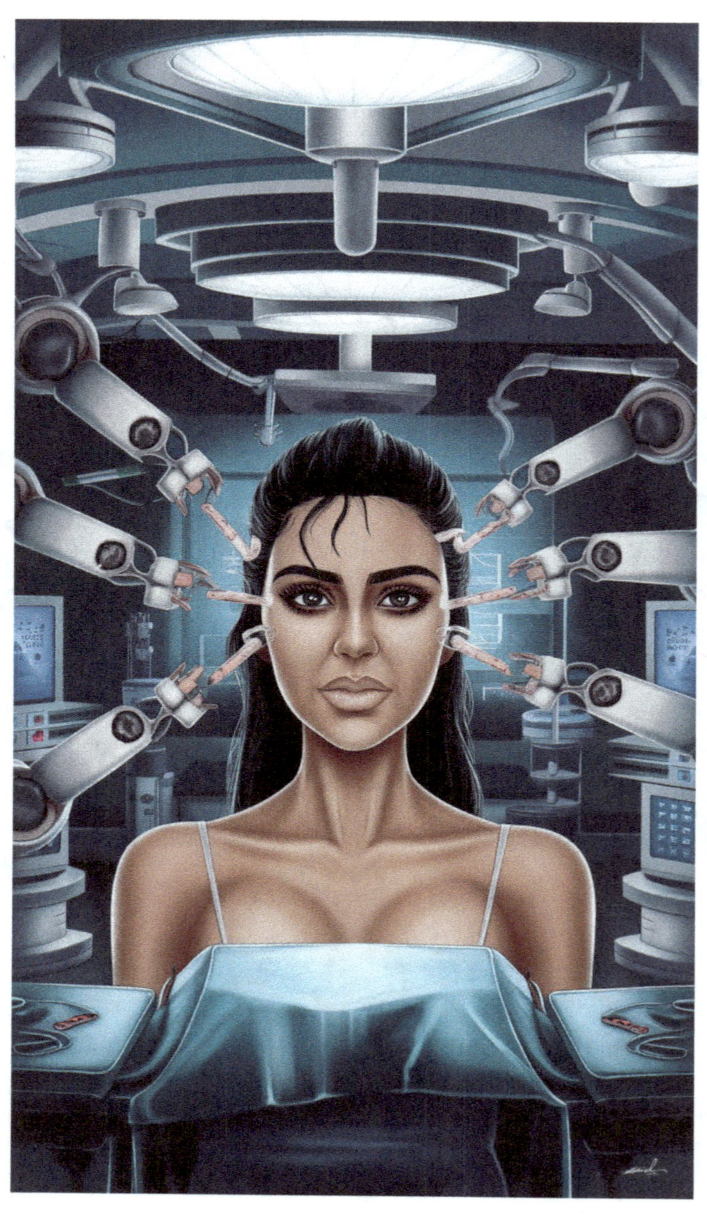

The Making of Kim Kardashian

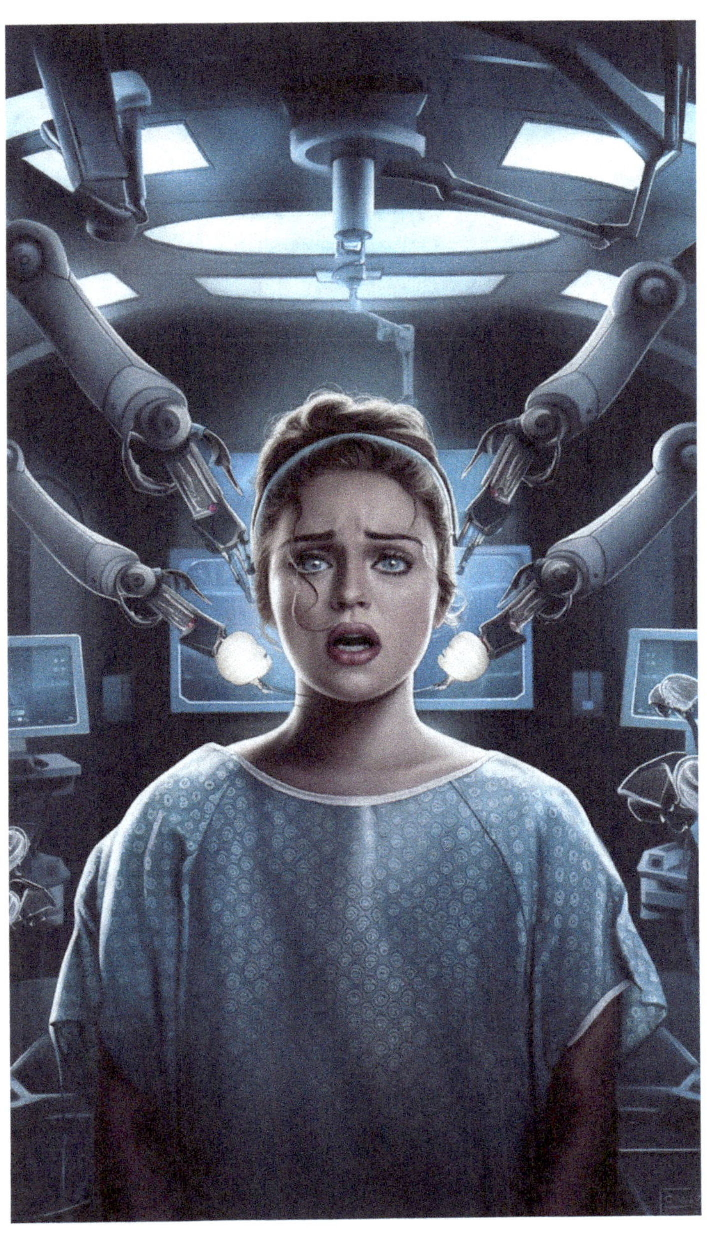

Lana Del Rey's Vocal Odyssey

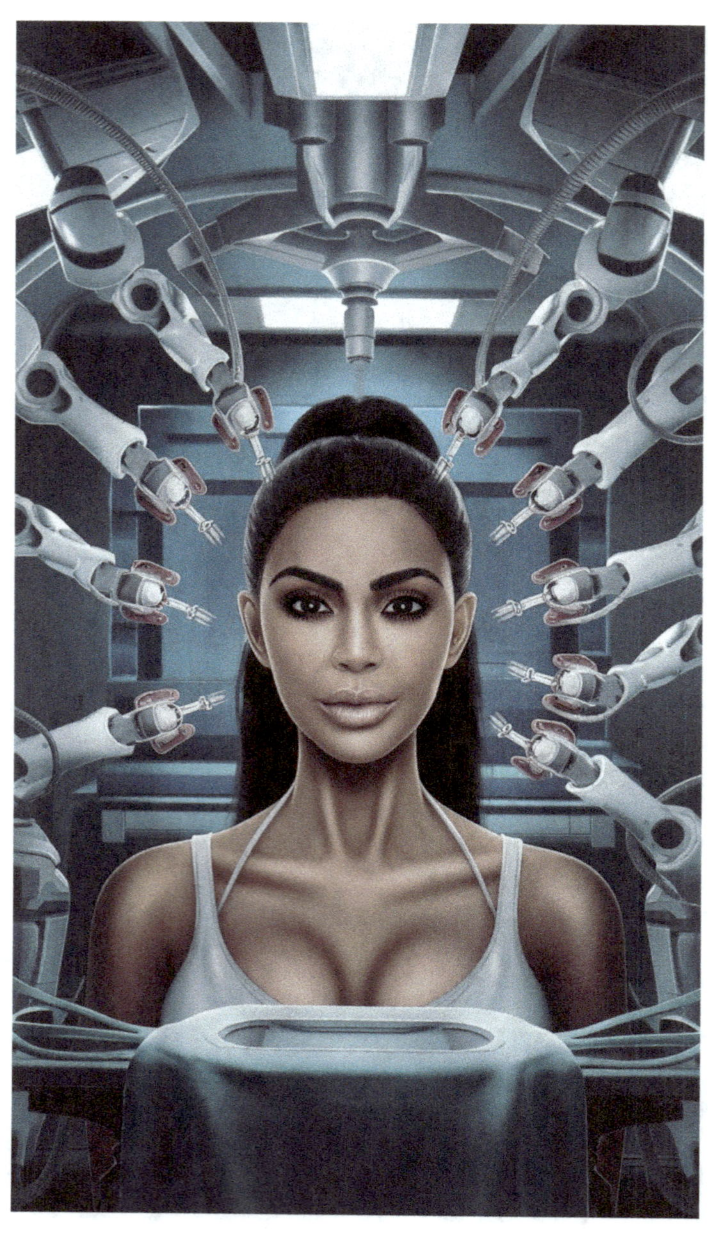

Sculpting Kim Kardashian

Celebrities and the elite are taking cosmetic enhancements to new extremes in their quest for physical perfection. Procedures like rib removal—which aims to create a slimmer waistline or a more dramatic hourglass figure—have been getting a lot of attention, even though they're pretty rare. Then there's toe shortening surgery, a peculiar yet sought-after option for those looking to make purely cosmetic changes to their feet.

Venturing deeper into the realm of unorthodox procedures, individuals are embracing forehead augmentation, dimpleplasty (also known as dimple surgery or dimple creation surgery), and calf reduction to sculpt their appearance according to societal ideals. The pursuit of perfection extends beyond physical features, with some celebrities like singer Adele who faced speculation about undergoing voice lift surgeries not only to enhance vocal performance, but also to modify their voice tone. Additionally, hand rejuvenation treatments and chin wing (jawline) surgeries exemplify the lengths individuals are willing to go to defy the signs of aging or conform to beauty standards.

However, as celebrities go through these amazing transformations, their once-familiar features get hidden under layers of surgical enhancements. Over-the-top cheek implants and unnaturally plumped lips take over their faces, serving as clear reminders of the risks that come with relentlessly chasing perfection. These extreme changes warn us about the dangers of cosmetic enhancements, turning familiar faces into cautionary tales about the downsides of striving for impossible beauty standards.

Glamour on the Go: Botox and Fillers - Celebrities' Quick Fix for Timeless Radiance

In Hollywood, where every little flaw is magnified by the unforgiving spotlight, Botox and fillers have become the ultimate secret weapons for many celebrities battling the signs of aging. These non-surgical wonders offer a quick fix to smooth out wrinkles and keep that timeless glow without the need for invasive procedures. Botox, derived from the botulinum toxin, works by temporarily relaxing underlying muscles, erasing fine lines and wrinkles with precision. Meanwhile, dermal fillers—made from hyaluronic acid or collagen-stimulating substances—plump up areas where volume has been lost, restoring a youthful fullness to the face. It's almost like they've sipped from the mythical Fountain of Youth!

The appeal of these treatments isn't just in how they transform appearances, but also in how convenient they are. With minimal downtime and visible results you can get in a single lunch break, Botox and fillers have become the go-to for celebrities looking to keep their flawless look amid hectic schedules and endless public appearances. Whether they're on the red carpet or posting Instagram selfies, these non-surgical options help stars shine with youthful radiance at every turn, defying the passage of time with each injection.

However, it's not just the visible results that have made Botox and fillers a celebrity obsession. In recent years, there's been a cultural shift, with celebrities leading the way in normalizing cosmetic procedures and breaking down the stigma around them. Leading the charge are sisters Kim Kardashian and Kylie Jenner. Their open discussions about their experiences with Botox and fillers have sparked a revolution in the beauty industry. By sharing their journeys to maintain a youthful look, they've not only demystified these treatments but also encouraged a more accepting attitude toward them, both in the entertainment industry and beyond. In doing so, they've empowered countless people to embrace cosmetic enhancements as a form of self-expression and self-care, turning the pursuit of beauty into a celebration of individuality and confidence.

Despite their appeal, these treatments also have a darker side of side effects and health risks that celebrities often overlook in their relentless quest for perfection. Issues can range from mild discomfort and bruising at the injection site to more serious complications like infections, allergic reactions, and even tissue damage. The potential dangers of Botox and fillers shouldn't be underestimated. Plus, the long-term effects of repeated injections aren't fully understood yet, raising concerns about the cumulative damage they might cause to the skin and underlying tissues over time.

Recently, studies have shown that dermal fillers might not completely disappear over time as we once thought. Instead, they can move around in the face, which can lead to that overfilled look some people call "pillow face." Evidence is coming out showing that fillers can shift to different areas, raising concerns about long-term effects. This has started conversations about how fillers are used and the importance of moderation to avoid unexpected changes in appearance.

Even with these risks, celebrities still line up at cosmetic clinics, chasing that elusive promise of eternal youth. Thanks to quick results and minimal downtime, Botox and fillers have become the go-to solutions for maintaining a flawless look in the fast-paced world of fame and fortune. But as the quest for perfection keeps escalating, it's important for both celebrities and the public to weigh the potential risks against the rewards and make informed choices about their beauty treatments. After all, true radiance comes from within, and no amount of Botox or fillers can replace the glow of genuine self-confidence and self-love.

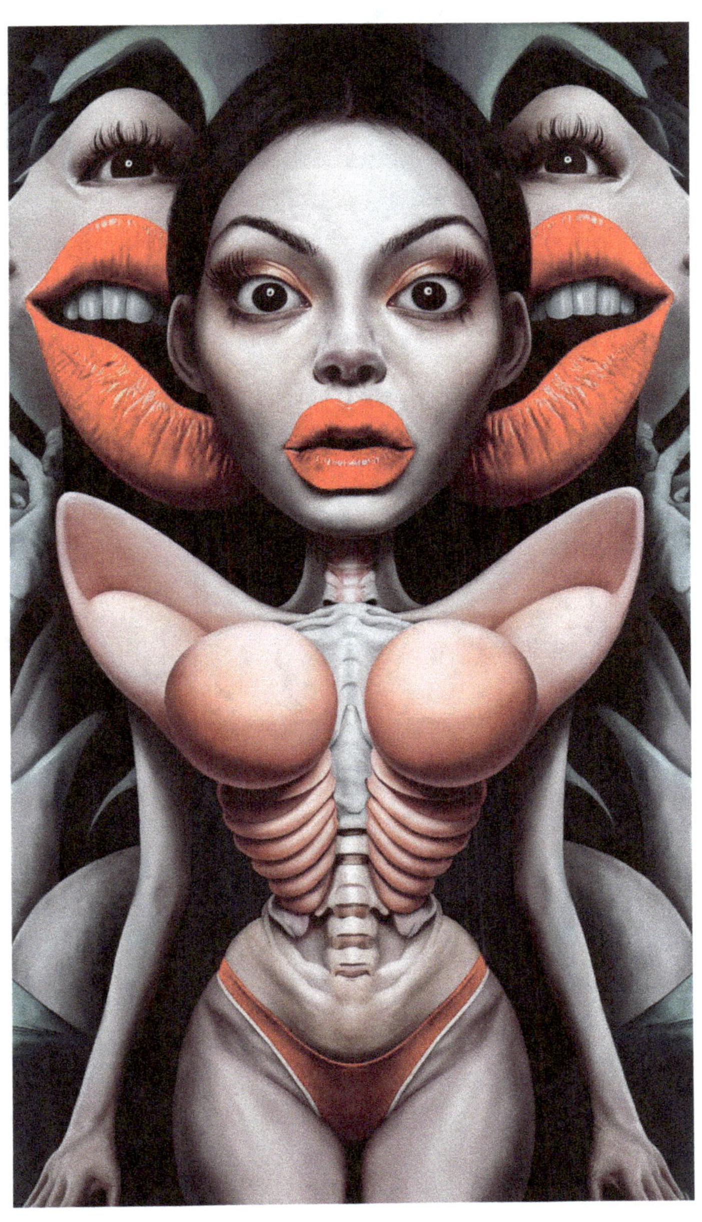

Ribs of Desire, Lips of Excess

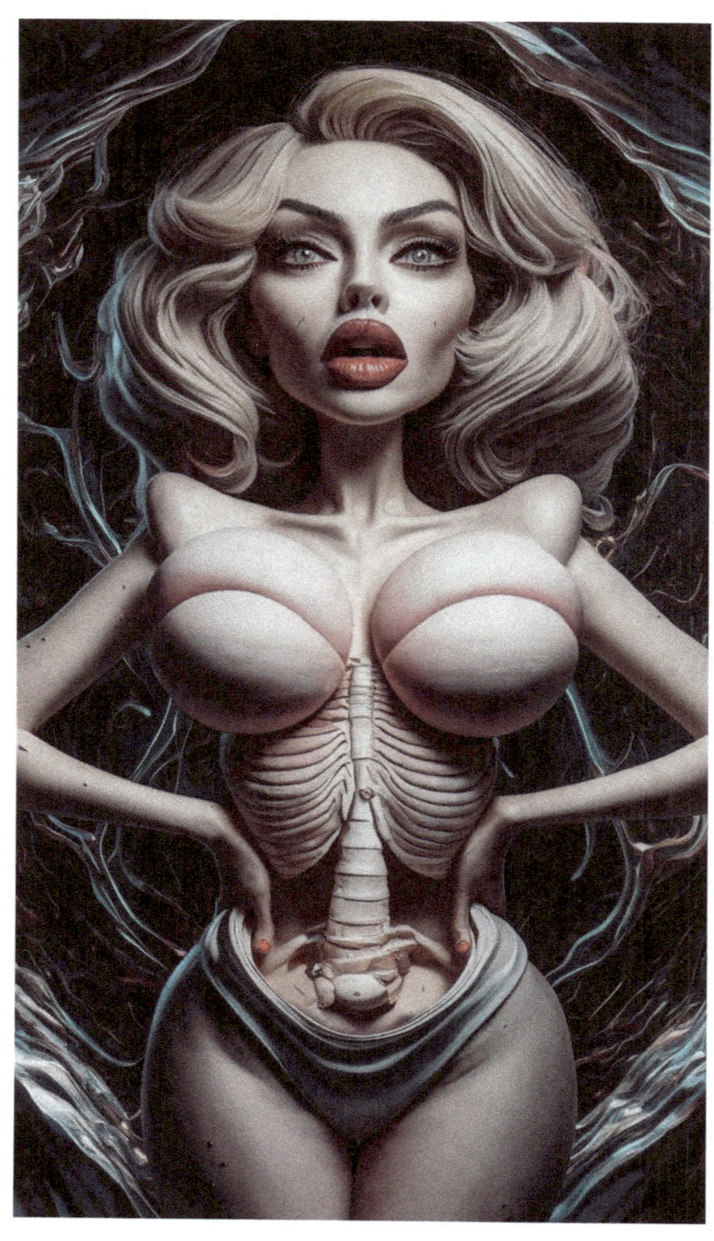

Anatomy of Artificial Beauty

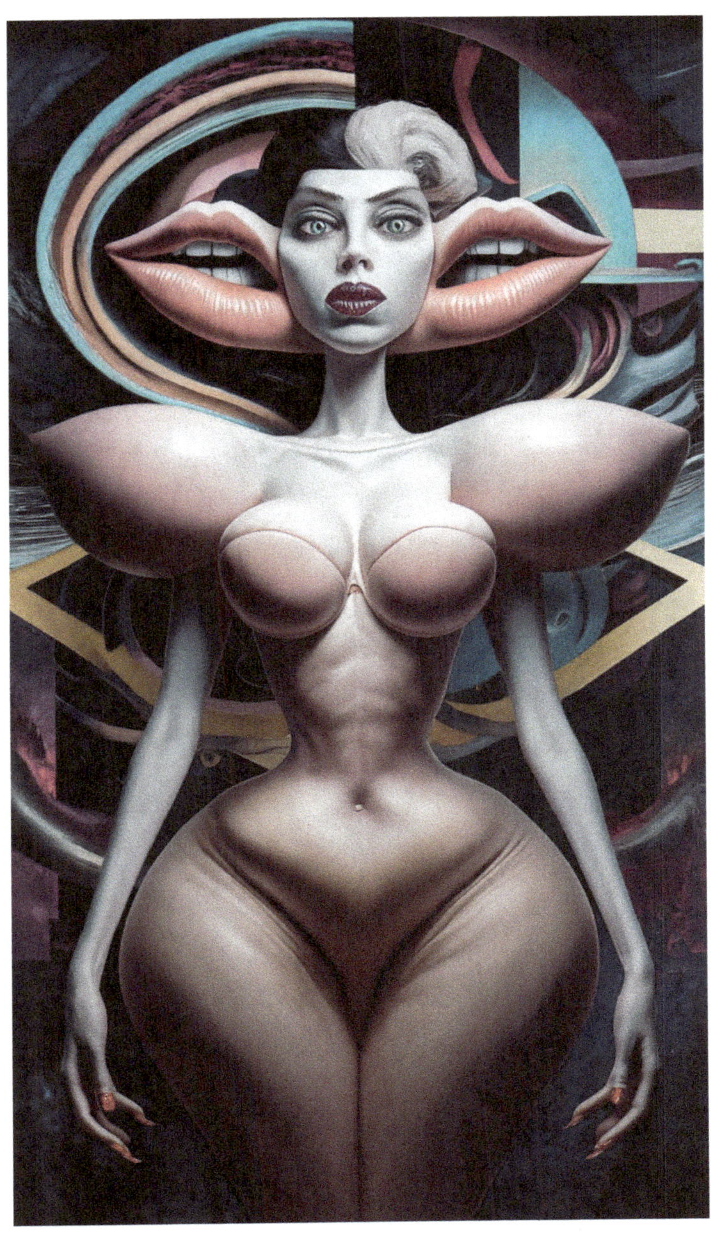

Body of Dreams

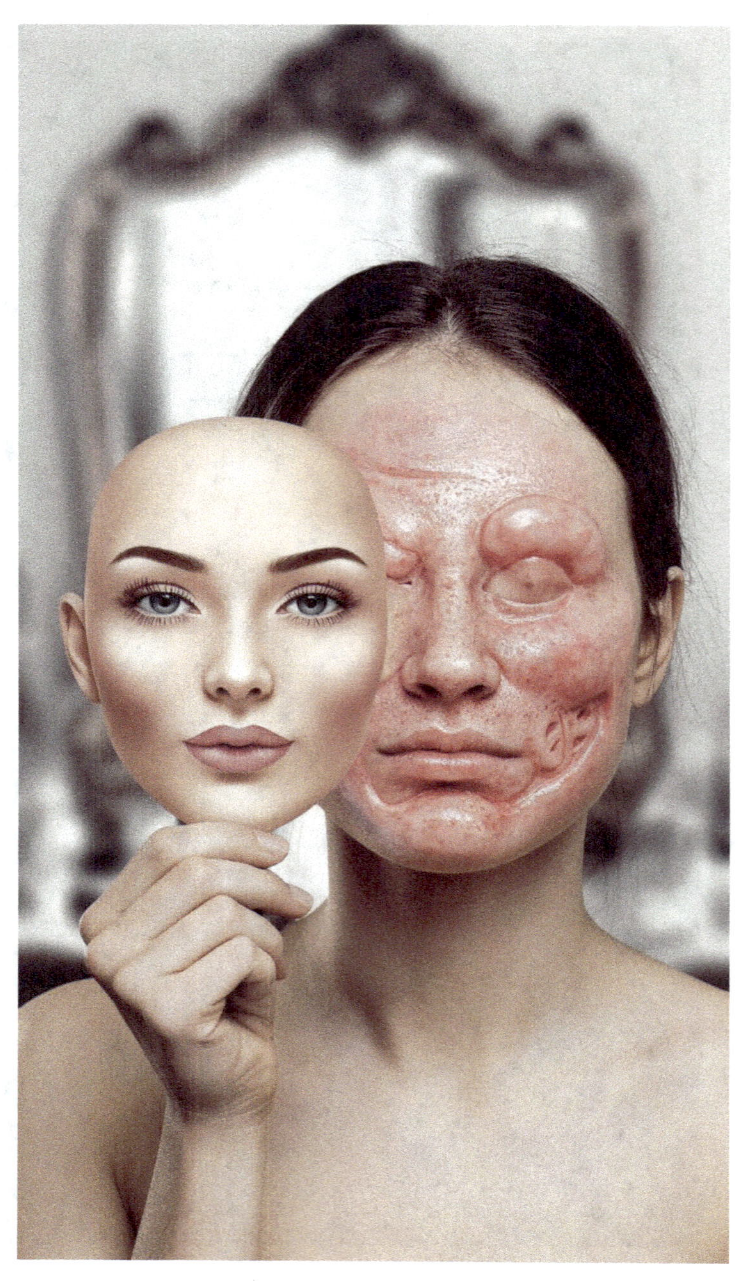

The Illusion of Beauty

Among the elite, rumors persist about secret clinics offering miraculous blood transfusions as a way to fight aging. While solid proof of these places remains elusive, intriguing stories continue to surface about celebrities and others exploring unconventional methods for staying youthful.

One well-known example is Ambrosia, a startup that made headlines for offering blood plasma infusions to older clients in the hopes of boosting vitality. Though it attracted significant attention and interest, Ambrosia eventually came under regulatory scrutiny. Following a cautionary warning from the FDA about its unproven practices, the company was forced to shut down.

Amidst the mystery, there are reports suggesting that high-profile figures may be involved in similar anti-aging pursuits. Rumors about tech mogul Elon Musk's interest in longevity research fuel speculation about his potential connections to experimental anti-aging treatments. Likewise, Hollywood icon Tom Cruise is occasionally mentioned in discussions about unconventional health practices, adding another layer to the intrigue.

Peter Thiel, a billionaire entrepreneur and co-founder of PayPal, has become a subject of intrigue due to his reputed interest in radical life extension. While his ventures in anti-aging research stir curiosity, the extent of his personal involvement remains shrouded in secrecy.

Rumors occasionally swirl around celebrities like Oprah Winfrey and Madonna, linking them to secret clinics and experimental anti-aging treatments. However, without solid evidence, these whispers remain speculative, reflecting society's ongoing fascination with the elusive quest for eternal youth.

Eternal Pursuits: Billionaires' Battle for Immortality

In Silicon Valley, where innovation and ambition go hand in hand, a new obsession has taken hold among tech giants: the pursuit of eternal life. While some dismiss the idea of defying mortality, others, like Jeff Bezos and Mark Zuckerberg, see it as a mission worth pouring millions into.

At the heart of California's tech hub, Bezos, the visionary behind Amazon, has turned his attention to the cutting-edge field of aging research. In 2021, he invested in Altos Labs, a biotech startup focused on cellular rejuvenation. With every dollar invested, Bezos fuels the possibility of a future where aging can be reversed, potentially resetting the clock with a simple tweak to our genes.

Bezos isn't alone in the battle against aging. Mark Zuckerberg, the mastermind behind Facebook, is right there with him, using his immense wealth to fight the effects of time. Through the Breakthrough Prize, which he co-founded with his wife Priscilla Chan, Zuckerberg supports the brilliant minds pushing the boundaries of longevity science. Their annual $3 million award acts as a beacon, encouraging scientists to uncover new breakthroughs in the quest to slow down or even reverse the aging process.

While others chase the dream of extending life, one figure stands apart: Elon Musk. The visionary behind Tesla and SpaceX, Musk dismisses the idea of prolonging human lifespans. To him, the pursuit of immortality isn't a triumph, but a potential tragedy— leading to stagnation and a world where progress halts, trapped by minds unwilling to change. While Bezos and Zuckerberg invest in the future of longevity, Musk stays firm in his belief that the real innovation lies not in preserving life, but in the limitless potential of minds free from the constraints of time.

As the quest for immortality continues, fueled by billions and driven by bold ambitions, one thing is clear: in the halls of Silicon Valley, where science and science fiction often merge, the pursuit of eternal life is no longer just a distant dream—it's a promise waiting to be realized.

Defying Destiny: The Silicon Valley Quest for Immortality

Within the heart of Silicon Valley, where innovation has no limits and the future feels like a blank canvas, aging isn't something to be accepted. Instead, it's questioned, dissected, and reimagined. In this world shaped by tech giants, aging is seen as a problem to solve—a code waiting to be cracked, with death itself viewed as a mere glitch in the system, just waiting to be fixed.

Leading the charge in the fight against aging is Peter Thiel, the enigmatic co-founder of PayPal and Palantir, and a pioneer in big data analytics. With vast resources and even bigger ambitions, Thiel has invested millions into anti-aging research, his focus set on a future where "90 is the new 50" by 2030. Through the Methuselah Foundation—a non-profit named after the biblical figure who lived for centuries—Thiel imagines a world where age is just a number, one that can be manipulated and controlled by the power of science.

For Thiel, the merging of advanced computing with biological breakthroughs offers the promise of a new era—one where human diseases are no different from software bugs, easily detected and fixed. In his view, even death will eventually lose its mystery, reduced to a problem waiting to be solved by human ingenuity and intellect.

Fueled by his desire for extended life, Thiel is one of the most outspoken advocates for anti-aging therapies, willing to push the limits of convention in his pursuit of immortality. One experiment that has particularly caught his attention is both fascinating and eerie: aged mice receiving transfusions of blood from their younger counterparts showed signs of partial rejuvenation in their muscles, brains, and organs. While the exact mechanisms behind this process remain unclear, scientists are working tirelessly to understand it, with the hope of one day using it to combat age-related diseases like dementia.

Even as Thiel and his peers push the boundaries of what's possible, their journey toward eternal youth hasn't been without controversy. Some ventures have crossed into bizarre territory, offering young blood transfusions to those willing to pay sky-high prices. However, the US Food and Drug Administration (FDA) quickly stepped in, questioning the effectiveness of such procedures and issuing a stern reminder that, despite its breakthroughs, science can still fall victim to misguided ambition.

As the quest for immortality plays out against the backdrop of Silicon Valley, one thing is clear: in this land of bold ideas and boundless ambition, where the line between reality and fiction fades a little more each day, the pursuit of eternal life isn't just a dream—it's a destiny waiting to be realized.

The Pursuit of Immortality: Inside Bryan Johnson's Quest for Eternal Youth

At the crossroads of scientific discovery and bold ambition, where the boundaries between reality and fiction fade, one man leads a daring experiment—an effort to uncover the elusive secret of eternal youth.

Meet Bryan Johnson, the millionaire trailblazer on a unique mission—to turn back the clock on aging. With vast resources and an unbounded vision, Johnson has committed an astonishing $2 million annually to the bold pursuit of bio-hacking his body, aiming to reverse the aging process. His journey is fueled by an unwavering determination to defy time itself.

In an exclusive interview with TIME, Johnson unveiled the details of his unconventional routine, revealing a regimen that would leave even seasoned bio-hackers in awe. His daily ritual includes swallowing 111 pills, wearing a health monitoring device on his penis to track nighttime erections, and donning a baseball cap that emits a red glow into his scalp. All of these steps are part of his ambitious plan to unlock the secrets of eternal youth.

Johnson's pursuit of youth goes far beyond supplements and monitoring. He's embraced the latest advancements in medical science, turning to an anti-aging algorithm to manage his body's functions. For him, this isn't just a fight against time—it's a war against his own "rascal mind." His mission is to push past the limits of mortality and recapture the vitality of youth.

With the dedication of a modern-day alchemist, Johnson spares no expense in his quest to reverse aging.

His routine includes blood transfusions with his teenage son, a daily intake of over 100 supplements, and an entire team of 30 doctors conducting regular body scans and MRIs. Every detail is carefully planned, each step bringing him closer to his elusive goal of turning back the clock.

For Johnson, mornings don't start with the usual routine but with his "green giant" smoothie, packed with ingredients aimed at revitalization and longevity. Collagen, spermidine, and creatine are just a few of the key components in his recipe for eternal youth, designed to nourish his body from the inside out.

Johnson's bold endeavors have caught the attention of powerful circles. Bloomberg spotlighted his ambitious mission, calling it "Project Blueprint," a reflection of the meticulous planning and unwavering determination that drive him closer to his ultimate goal of reversing the aging process.

As the world watches closely, Bryan Johnson's journey unfolds like a modern-day odyssey—one filled with ambition, sacrifice, and an unyielding pursuit of immortality. His quest reflects a timeless truth: the desire for eternity, the drive to challenge the very limits of existence, and the belief that with enough determination and daring, even time itself can be conquered.

Outside the boundaries of traditional medicine lies a world of experimental treatments and unproven elixirs, all promising to unlock the secret to eternal youth. Celebrities and elites dive into untested supplements, vitamin cocktails, controversial hormone therapies, and stem cell injections, sparing no cost in their pursuit. Some even explore more contentious options like human growth hormone (HGH) injections or vampire facials (platelet-rich plasma therapy). Though these treatments boast rejuvenating effects, they often carry risks and uncertain outcomes.

One well-known example of an untested supplement often associated with the fountain of youth is human growth hormone (HGH). Naturally produced by the pituitary gland, HGH plays a key role in growth, metabolism, and cell repair. It has gained attention as a potential anti-aging treatment due to its ability to promote tissue growth, increase muscle mass, and reduce body fat. However, despite its popularity, the effectiveness and safety of HGH for anti-aging purposes remain areas of ongoing debate and research.

Some advocates of HGH argue that supplementing with this hormone can reverse the visible signs of aging, such as wrinkles, sagging skin, and reduced energy levels. They believe that HGH injections have the potential to rejuvenate the body, giving it a more youthful appearance while also boosting overall health and vitality. However, these claims are often met with skepticism, as the long-term effects and risks of HGH supplementation are not fully understood.

Despite its popularity, the use of HGH as an anti-aging treatment remains controversial, with its effectiveness and safety still uncertain. Clinical studies on HGH supplementation in older adults have produced mixed results. While some research has shown modest improvements in body composition and physical function, other studies have found little to no significant benefits. This uncertainty continues to fuel debates about whether HGH is a truly effective tool in the fight against aging.

Additionally, HGH supplementation comes with serious risks. Side effects can include fluid retention, joint pain, and carpal tunnel syndrome, as well as an increased risk of diabetes and cardiovascular disease. It can also disrupt the body's natural hormone balance, potentially leading to long-term health complications. These dangers highlight the importance of weighing the risks carefully before considering HGH as an anti-aging treatment.

Even with the known risks, HGH continues to be marketed as a "fountain of youth" by some anti-aging clinics and supplement manufacturers, targeting individuals searching for quick solutions to aging concerns. However, it's crucial for consumers to approach this with caution and consult healthcare professionals before considering HGH supplementation, as its use comes with significant risks and uncertainties. Making informed decisions is essential when dealing with treatments that could pose serious health consequences.

Glowing with Celestial Youth: The Allure of Vampire Facials

Vampire facials, also known as platelet-rich plasma (PRP) therapy, have become popular for their rejuvenating effects, especially among celebrities looking to maintain youthful skin. This cosmetic treatment involves drawing a small amount of the patient's blood, usually from the arm, and processing it to separate the platelet-rich plasma. This plasma, packed with growth factors and proteins believed to aid in tissue repair and regeneration, is then either injected into the face or applied topically after micro-needling for enhanced absorption.

The micro-needling process involves using a device with fine needles to create tiny punctures in the skin's surface. These micro-injuries trigger the body's natural healing response, encouraging collagen production and skin renewal. When paired with the application of platelet-rich plasma, vampire facials are said to improve skin texture, tone, and overall appearance. This combination is believed to reduce signs of aging such as fine lines, wrinkles, and uneven pigmentation, offering a more youthful look.

Vampire facials have gained significant media attention and popularity among beauty enthusiasts, largely due to their association with celebrities. Kim Kardashian famously shared her vampire facial experience on social media, which sparked widespread interest in the treatment. Other celebrities rumored to have tried the procedure include model Bar Refaeli and actress Angelina Jolie, among others, further fueling the buzz around this rejuvenating skincare trend.

Despite its popularity, vampire facials remain a topic of debate, with some medical professionals questioning both their effectiveness and safety. While supporters highlight the potential benefits for skin rejuvenation, skeptics point out that more research is needed to back these claims and ensure the procedure's safety, especially when done by unqualified practitioners. As with any cosmetic treatment, it's crucial for individuals considering vampire facials to consult with a qualified healthcare provider to discuss the risks, benefits, and whether the treatment suits their specific needs.

However, it's often the most extravagant claims that captivate the public—the whispered rumors of secret labs creating miracle potions and serums from exotic ingredients. Stories of celebrities traveling to remote corners of the world in search of the ultimate anti-aging remedy continue to circulate, sparking both fascination and speculation.

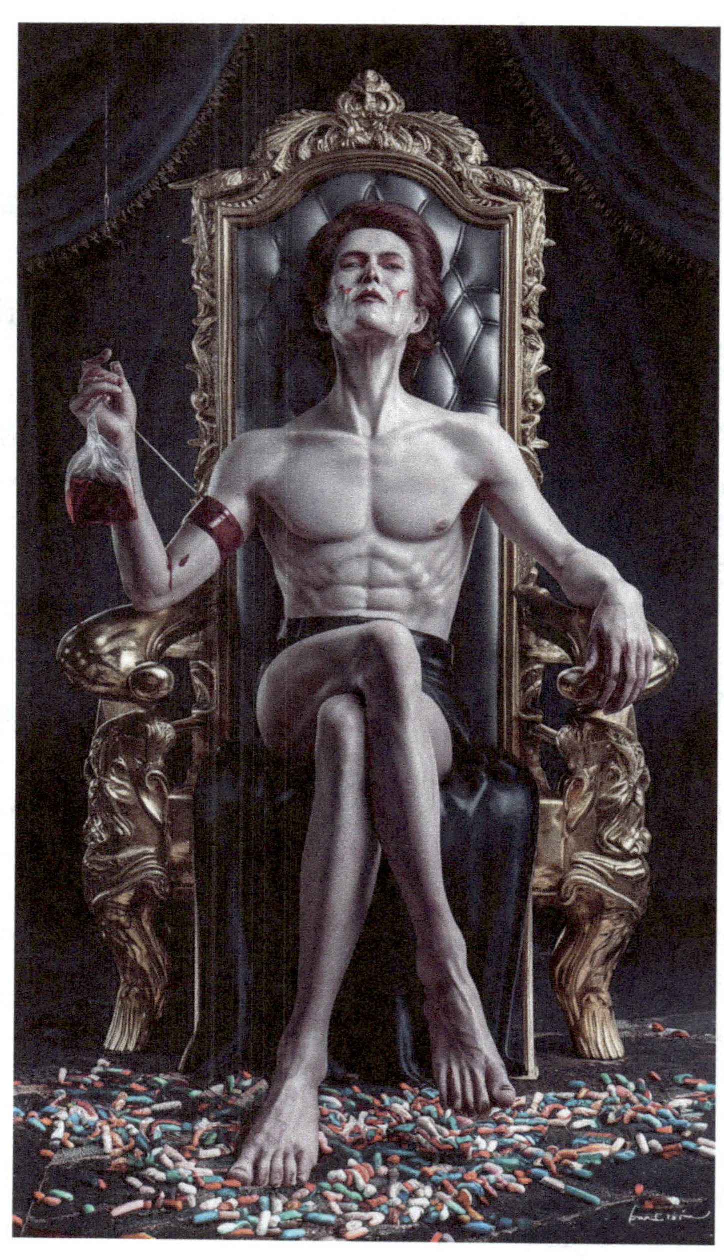

Bloodlines of Vanity

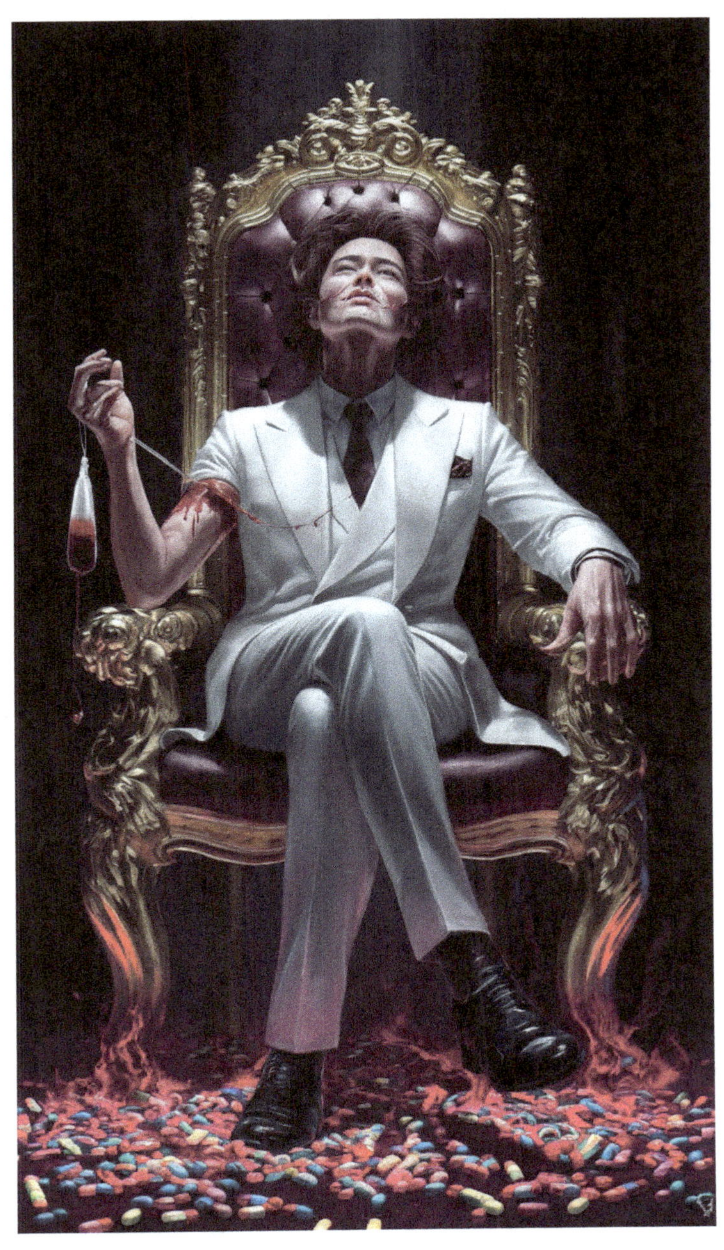

King of Blood and Pills

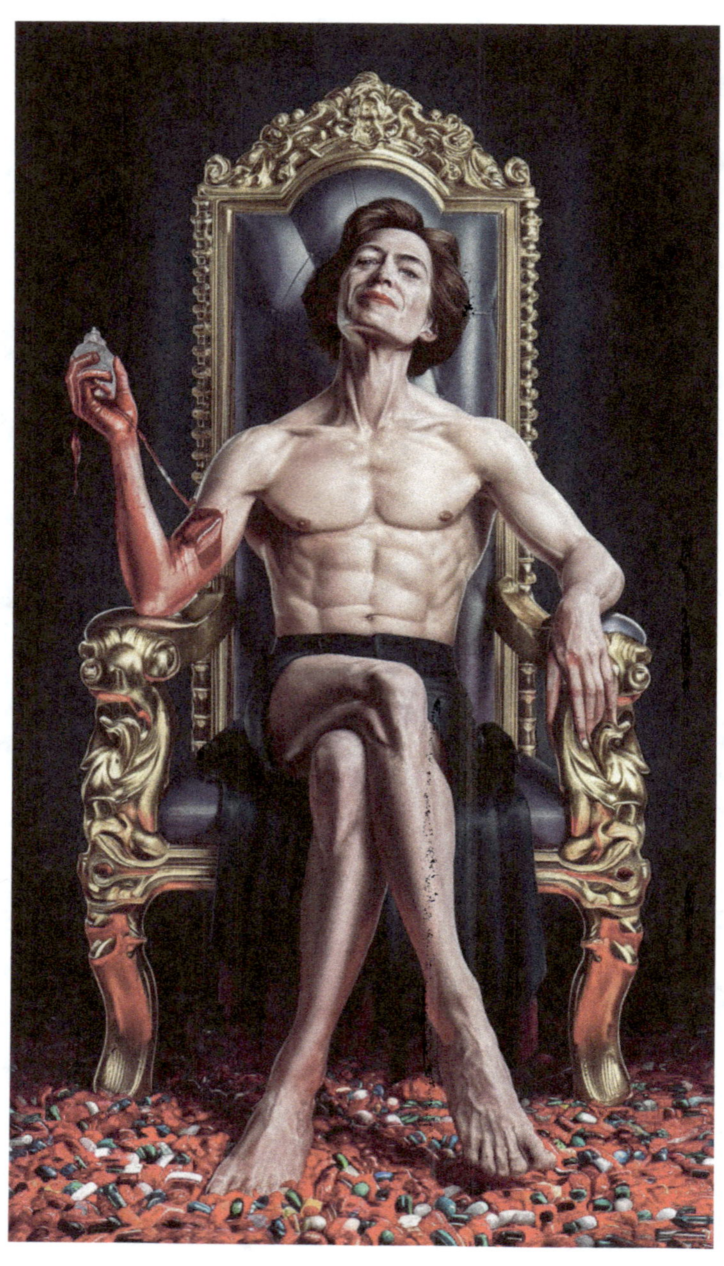

Reign of the Ageless

Beneath the surface of anti-aging treatments lies a shadowy side—clandestine laboratories cloaked in secrecy and whispered about for their supposed miraculous elixirs. Hidden from public view and beyond the reach of regulatory oversight, these labs are rumored to be centers of experimentation, creating serums and potions from exotic ingredients in the endless quest for eternal youth.

Even with their mysterious nature, rumors of clandestine laboratories capture the public's imagination, adding to the allure of the forbidden and the promise of extraordinary rejuvenation. These rumors often stem from speculation, tabloid gossip, and conspiracy theories, spinning tales of hidden facilities where age-defying potions and elixirs are secretly brewed.

The potions and serums reportedly created in these secretive laboratories are said to be made from exotic ingredients gathered from far-flung locations and obscure sources. These ingredients, which range from rare botanical extracts to unusual animal-derived substances, are believed to hold the secrets to everlasting youth and vitality.

Celebrities on Anti-Aging Pilgrimages: Madonna and Gywneth Paltrow

Fame and fortune often fuel an unrelenting pursuit of eternal youth. Renowned figures like Madonna and Gwyneth Paltrow have captured headlines for their rumored searches for the ultimate anti-aging elixir, embarking on journeys to distant parts of the world in search of ancient wisdom and natural remedies.

Madonna's Mystical Journeys

Madonna, a global icon known for her ageless beauty, has long been rumored to seek out unconventional anti-aging remedies inspired by various cultural traditions. Reports suggest that she has traveled to remote locations, exploring the secrets of Ayurveda in India and participating in traditional healing ceremonies deep within the Amazon rainforest. While the details of Madonna's journey remain largely unknown, her commitment to exploring ancient healing practices highlights the allure of exotic destinations in the quest for everlasting youth.

Gwyneth Paltrow's Wellness Quest

Similarly, Gwyneth Paltrow, founder of the holistic lifestyle brand Goop, has delved into unconventional wellness practices in her search for eternal youth. Rumors suggest she has traveled to renowned wellness retreats tucked away in the Himalayas and luxurious resorts along the shores of Bali. Whether experiencing Ayurvedic therapies or exploring ancient healing practices, Paltrow's rumored quest for anti-aging solutions reflects the growing interest in alternative wellness practices and the appeal of global exploration in the pursuit of beauty and vitality.

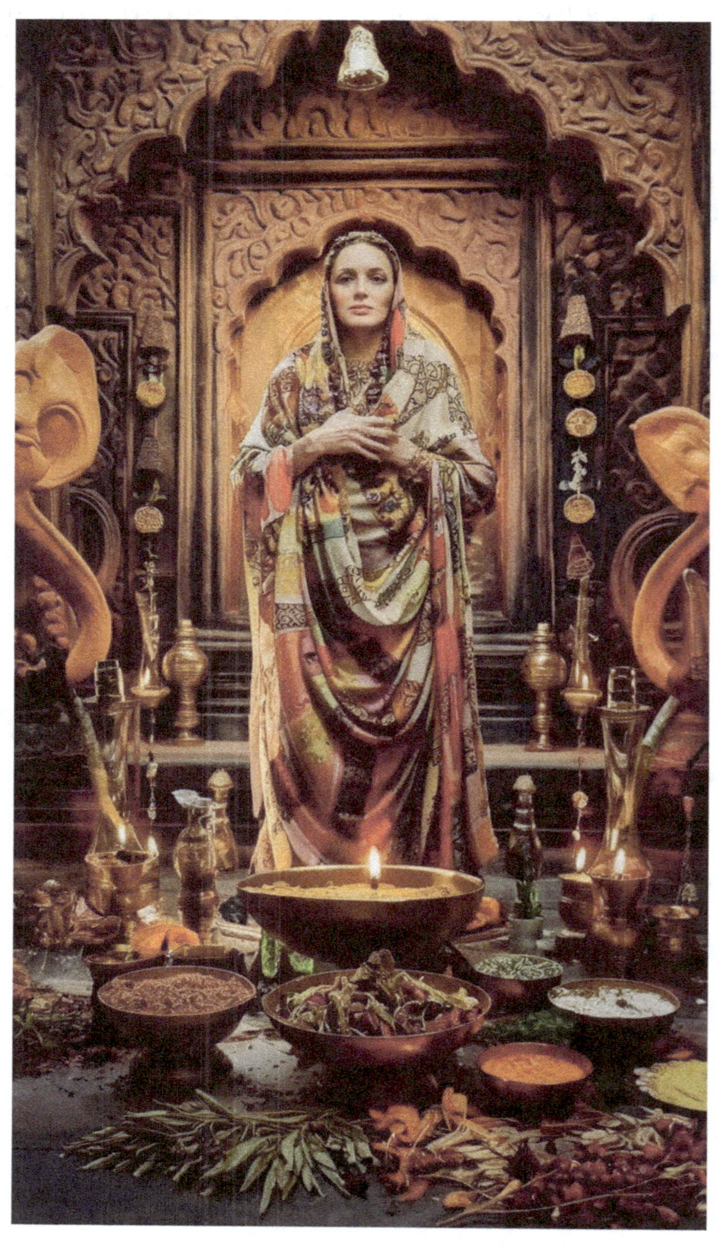

Madonna: Ancient Wisdom, Modern Vanity

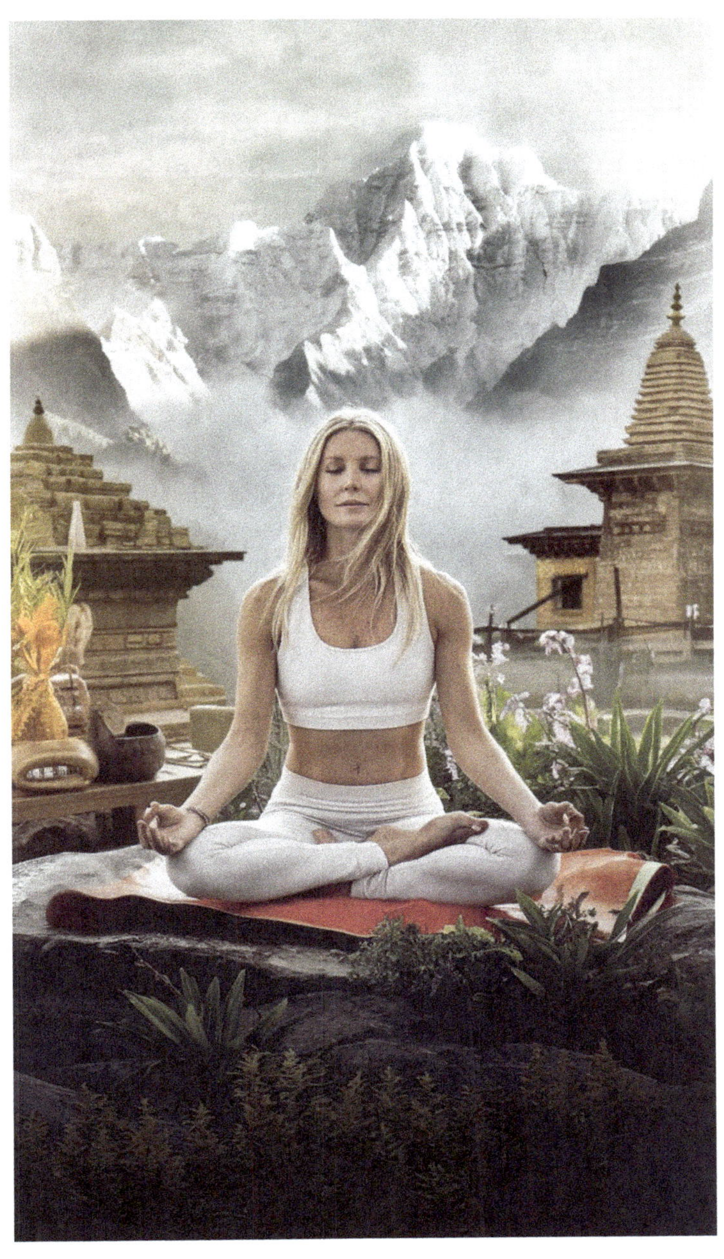

Gwyneth Paltrow's Path to Agelessness

Celebrities, always striving for the perfect physique, are no strangers to extreme and controversial diets. From lemon juice cleanses to the bizarre practice of tapeworm ingestion, these diets promise rapid weight loss but carry significant risks and fuel heated debates. This section delves into the intriguing intersection of fame and fad diets, spotlighting ten of the most notorious dietary crazes that have captured headlines and raised questions about their safety and effectiveness. Driven by the pursuit of physical perfection, celebrities often lead the way in embracing these methods. From Hollywood icons to pop stars, the appeal of quick-fix diets spans the entertainment industry. In these pages, we explore the rumored connections between famous figures and some of the most infamous dieting trends in recent history.

The Master Cleanse (Lemon Detox Diet): The Master Cleanse, also known as the Lemon Detox Diet, became popular for its promise of detoxifying the body through a simple mixture of lemon juice, maple syrup, cayenne pepper, and water. While proponents praise its cleansing effects, critics argue that its extreme calorie restriction and lack of essential nutrients make it a risky choice for weight loss. Among the celebrities rumored to have tried the Master Cleanse is Beyoncé. Reports suggest she turned to this lemon-infused concoction to lose weight quickly for certain roles or events. Actor and musician Jared Leto has also been linked to the Master

Cleanse, further highlighting the diet's appeal among Hollywood's elite.

The Atkins Diet: The Atkins Diet made waves in the dieting world with its high-protein, low-carbohydrate approach, designed to induce ketosis for fat burning. While supporters praise its effectiveness, critics point out the potential risks, such as nutrient deficiencies, that can come with long-term adherence. Kim Kardashian has openly shared her experience with the Atkins Diet, crediting it for helping her shed weight after pregnancy. Similarly, Friends star Jennifer Aniston reportedly turned to the low-carb lifestyle to maintain her iconic figure amidst the demands of Hollywood.

The Cabbage Soup Diet: Supporters of the Cabbage Soup Diet claim it can help people lose weight quickly by consuming large amounts of cabbage soup over a seven-day period. However, nutritionists warn that its extreme calorie restriction and lack of nutritional balance raise concerns about both its sustainability and potential health risks. Buffy the Vampire Slayer star Sarah Michelle Gellar and My Name is Earl actress Jaime Pressly are both rumored to have tried the Cabbage Soup Diet. Whether they were aiming for a quick slim-down or were drawn to the appeal of a steaming bowl of greens, these Hollywood stars found themselves caught up in the cabbage craze.

The Baby Food Diet: The Baby Food Diet gained popularity among celebrities for its simplicity and portion control, replacing regular meals with jars of baby food. Despite its appeal, critics argue that the diet is impractical for adults and lacks the essential nutrients needed for overall health. Jennifer Aniston, known for her ageless beauty and youthful glow, has been linked to this trend, swapping out solid meals for jars of pureed foods. Joining her in the baby food craze is Legally Blonde star Reese Witherspoon, proving that even Hollywood royalty can be tempted by the allure of infant-sized portions.

The Tapeworm Diet: One of the most extreme and dangerous weight-loss methods, has fascinated and horrified people in Hollywood and beyond. This controversial approach involves ingesting tapeworm cysts or pills containing tapeworm eggs, with the goal of allowing the parasite to live in the digestive tract and consume food, supposedly aiding in weight loss. Although no specific celebrities have been definitively linked to the Tapeworm Diet, rumors persist about high-profile individuals experimenting with this risky practice in their pursuit of a slimmer figure.

The appeal of the Tapeworm Diet lies in its promise of effortless weight loss, as proponents claim the tapeworm reduces calorie absorption, leading to weight loss. However, the dangers far outweigh the benefits, with risks including severe nutritional deficiencies, gastrointestinal issues, and even life-threatening conditions such as intestinal obstruction or neurocysticercosis, a parasitic infection of the brain.

Even with its inherent risks, the Tapeworm Diet's allure has persisted, largely due to its secretive nature. The absence of confirmed celebrity endorsements keeps the diet shrouded in mystery, which only adds to its notorious reputation. As rumors of Hollywood's fascination with this extreme method continue to circulate, they serve as a stark reminder of the dangers associated with chasing quick-fix solutions. The Tapeworm Diet remains a cautionary tale, highlighting the risks of prioritizing physical perfection over health and well-being, and illustrating the extreme lengths some are willing to go to in their relentless pursuit of the ideal physique.

The Werewolf Diet (Lunar Diet): The Werewolf Diet, also known as the Lunar Diet, claims that fasting in alignment with the lunar calendar can help regulate metabolism and promote weight loss. Despite its mystical appeal, there is little scientific evidence to support its effectiveness, leaving many skeptical. Pop icon Madonna and actress Demi Moore have both been linked to the Lunar Diet, a regimen that aligns fasting with the phases of the moon. Whether motivated by a fascination with the moon or a quest for inner peace, these stars have embraced the allure of moonlit fasting.

The Alkaline Diet: Advocates of the Alkaline Diet claim that it can prevent diseases and promote weight loss by focusing on consuming alkalizing foods. However, critics argue that the diet's restrictive nature can limit essential nutrients, and there is a lack of scientific evidence to back up its health claims. Fashion icon Victoria Beckham and wellness enthusiast Gwyneth Paltrow have both been rumored to follow the Alkaline Diet, which emphasizes maintaining a pH-balanced eating regimen. From green juices to alkaline-rich foods, these celebrities have reportedly embraced this lifestyle in their quest for holistic health and vitality.

The Five-Bite Diet: As the name implies, the Five-Bite Diet limits individuals to consuming just five bites of food for both lunch and dinner, with breakfast completely omitted. While supporters highlight its simplicity and portion control, nutritionists warn against the dangers of extreme calorie restriction and the risk of nutrient deficiencies. Though there are few confirmed celebrity endorsements of the Five-Bite Diet, rumors swirl about unnamed stars adopting this minimalist approach to portion control.

The Breatharian Diet: The Breatharian Diet takes extreme dieting to unprecedented levels by promoting a lifestyle free of both food and water, claiming that air and sunlight are sufficient for sustenance. Despite its advocates, medical experts strongly warn of the severe risks of starvation and dehydration associated with this practice. In a light-hearted comment, actress Michelle Pfeiffer once joked about experimenting with "breatharianism," a diet supposedly fueled by nothing but air and sunlight. While her remarks were met with disbelief and amusement, they highlight the ongoing fascination with extreme dieting trends in celebrity circles.

The Grapefruit Diet: Rounding out our list is the Grapefruit Diet, which requires consuming grapefruit or grapefruit juice with every meal to supposedly boost fat-burning. While grapefruit is undoubtedly nutritious, providing vitamins and antioxidants, critics question its effectiveness for significant weight loss and raise concerns about its potential interactions with certain medications. Actress Brooke Shields and singer Kylie Minogue have both been rumored to have tried the Grapefruit Diet, which promotes the fat-burning properties of this citrus superfood. Whether drawn to the tangy sweetness of grapefruit or simply enticed by the allure of another diet trend, these stars have found themselves captivated by the promise of grapefruit-fueled weight loss.

Behind the glamour, however, lies a darker reality—potential health risks and questionable science often accompany these extreme and controversial diets. For this reason, it's essential to approach these trends with caution and skepticism, prioritizing evidence-based practices and consulting healthcare professionals to achieve healthy and sustainable weight management goals.

Exploring the Phenomenon of Ozempic Use for Weight Loss

In recent years, the pharmaceutical drug Ozempic has made headlines not for its original use in treating type 2 diabetes, but for its unexpected role as a weight loss aid. Initially developed to help diabetic patients manage blood sugar levels, Ozempic has gained the attention of celebrities and the public alike for its reported ability to suppress appetite and promote weight loss. This off-label use has sparked widespread interest, further blurring the lines between medical treatment and celebrity-fueled weight loss trends.

The Rise of Ozempic

Ozempic's shift from a diabetes treatment to a popular weight loss aid reflects the growing trend of pharmaceutical drugs being used for off-label purposes. While its primary role is to manage diabetes, its secondary benefits in weight loss have generated significant interest, particularly among those looking for a quick solution to shed pounds. The growing availability of Ozempic in beauty clinics—places typically reserved for Botox, fillers, and facials—raises concerns, especially as the increased demand for weight loss purposes has led to shortages, leaving diabetic patients struggling to access the medication they need. This trend highlights the ethical and medical dilemmas surrounding the use of medications beyond their intended purposes.

The growing popularity of Ozempic as a weight loss tool has been fueled in part by endorsements from high-profile celebrities like Adele, Rebel Wilson, Sharon Osbourne, and Elon Musk. Their public acknowledgment of using Ozempic as part of their weight loss journeys has pushed the drug into the spotlight, sparking widespread discussions about its effectiveness and safety for achieving dramatic transformations. These endorsements have not only boosted interest but also raised important questions about the potential risks involved in using a medication intended for diabetes management for off-label weight loss purposes.

Efficacy and Safety Concerns

Despite its rising popularity as a weight loss aid, questions remain about the long-term effectiveness and safety of Ozempic for individuals without diabetes. While some studies indicate that Ozempic can lead to significant weight loss in non-diabetic users, concerns linger over potential side effects and whether the weight loss achieved through pharmaceutical intervention alone is sustainable in the long run. These uncertainties highlight the need for further research and caution when considering Ozempic as a solution for weight management outside its intended use.

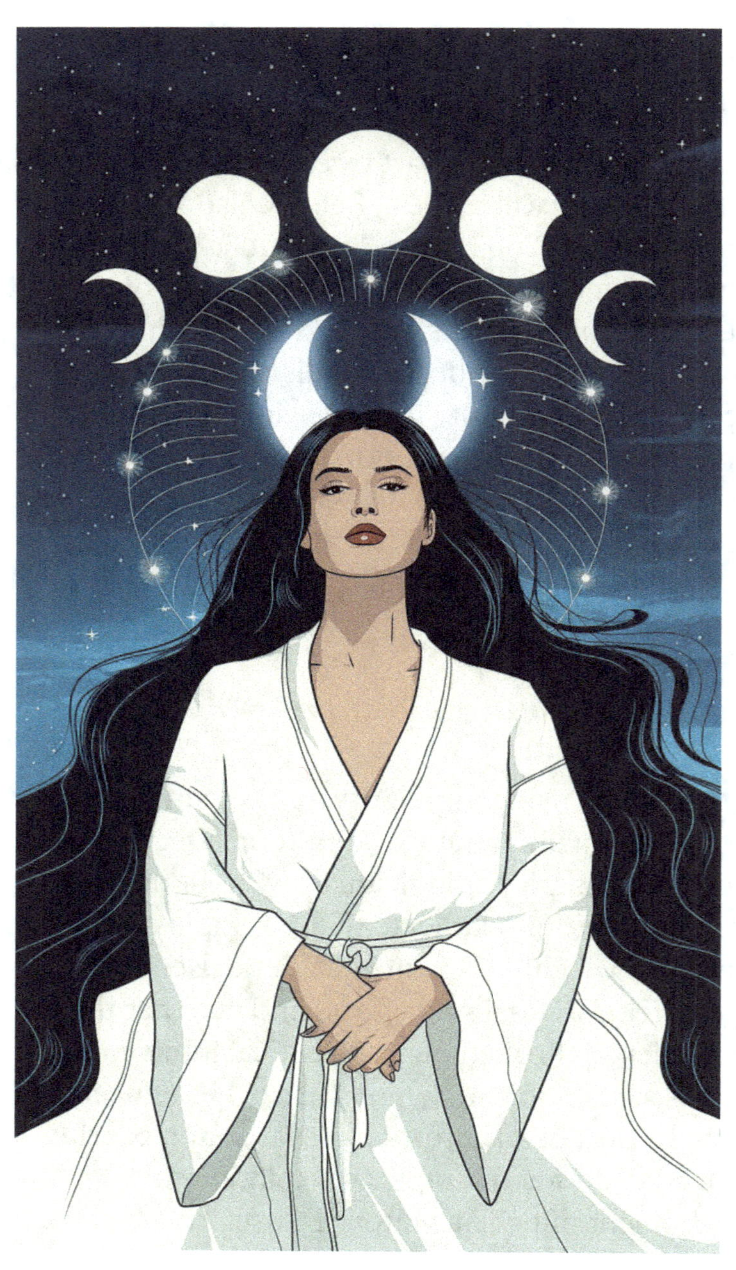

Demi Moore's Lunar Ritual

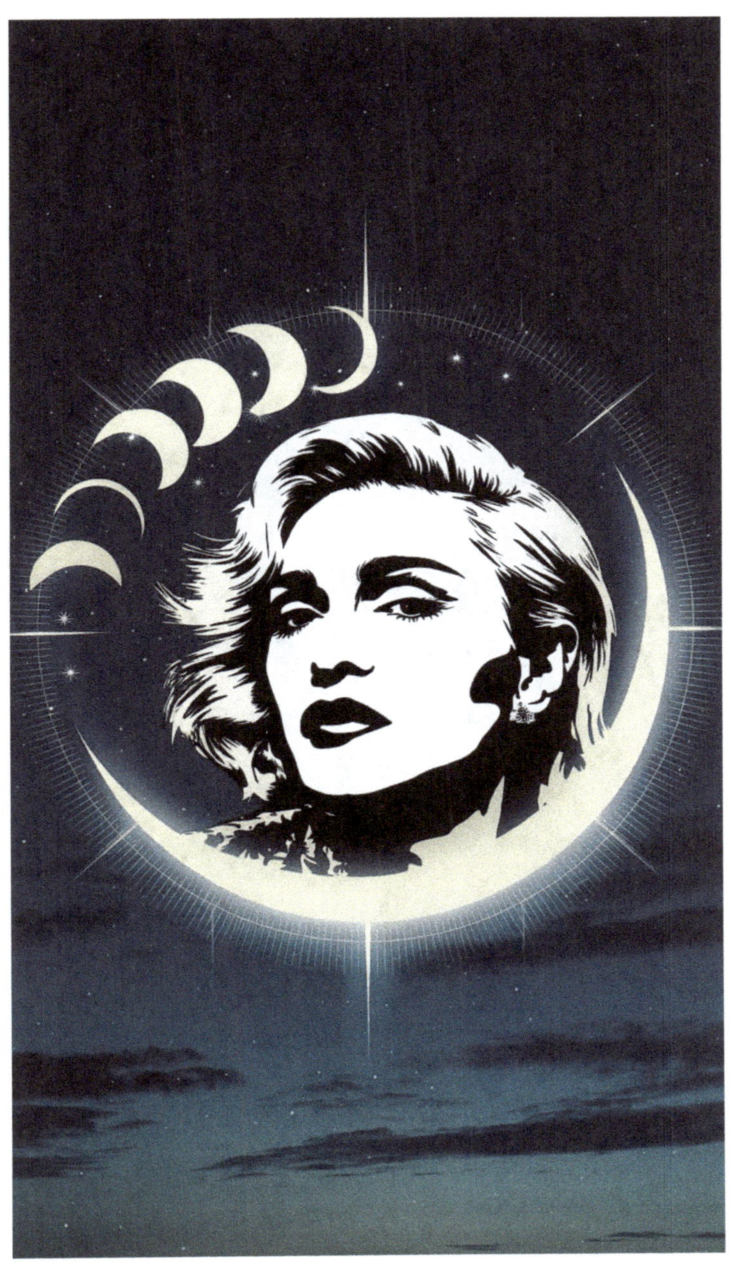

Madonna Illuminated by Lunar Reflections

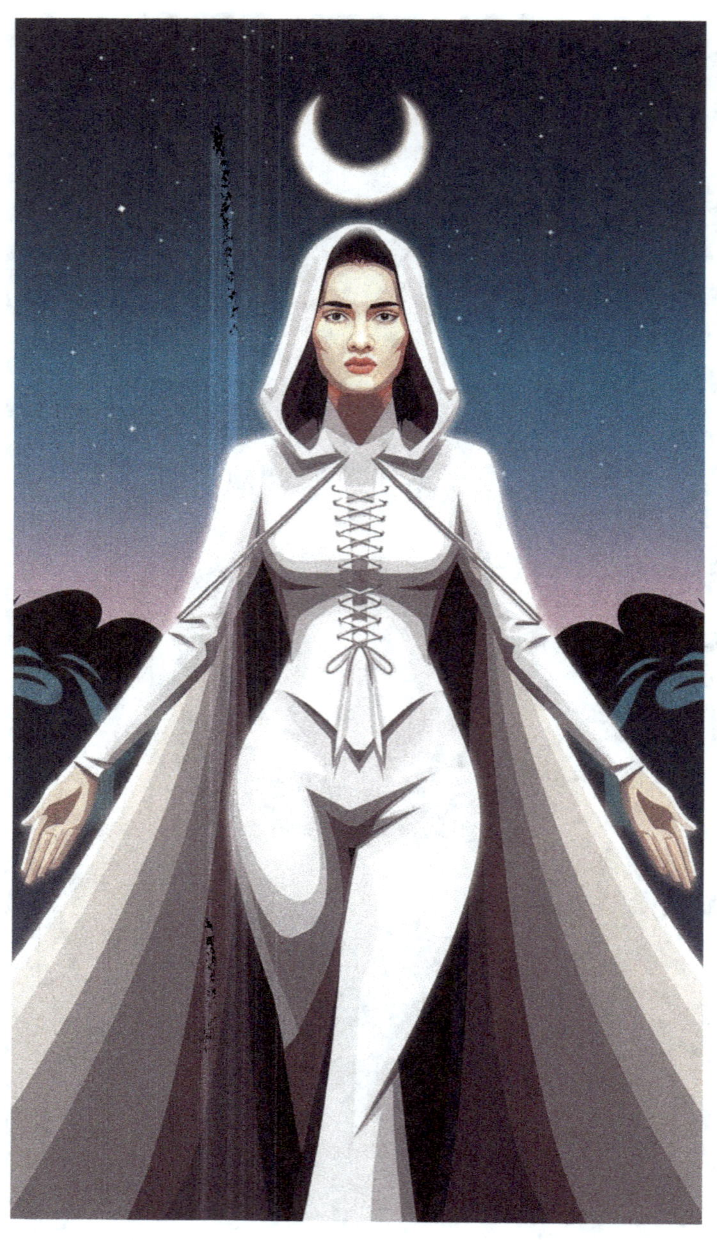

Madonna: A Dance with the Moon

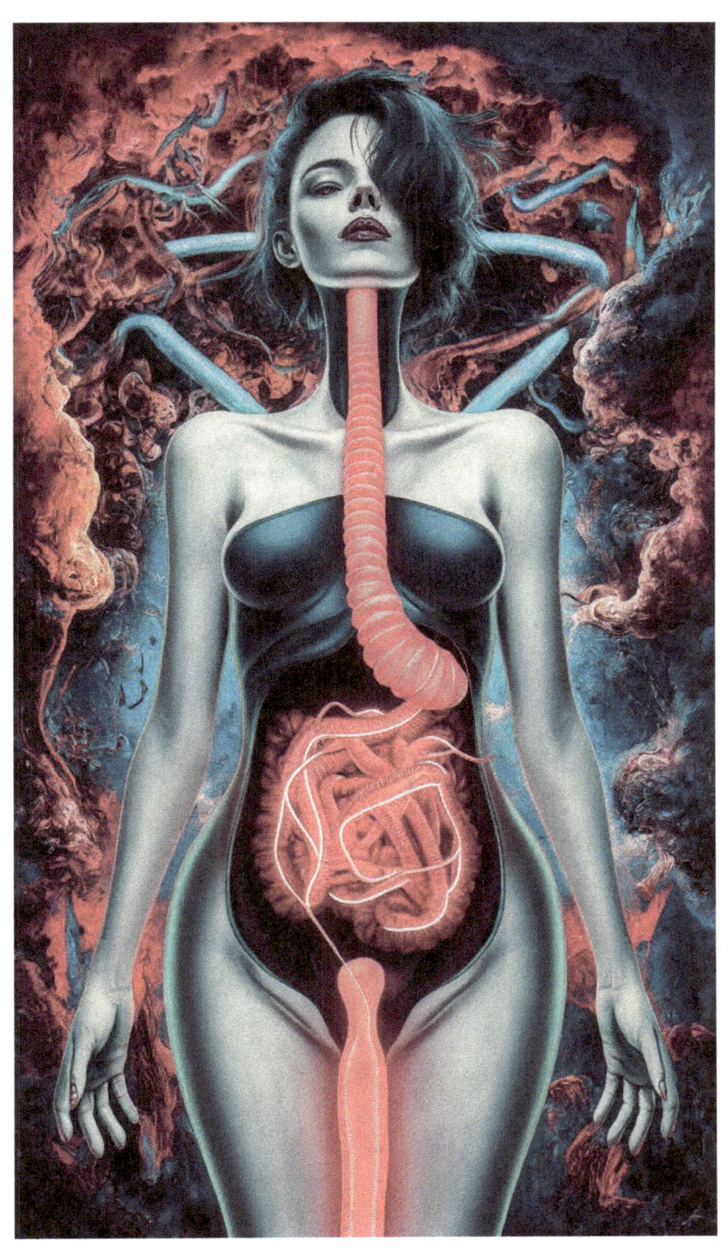

Parasite of Vanity

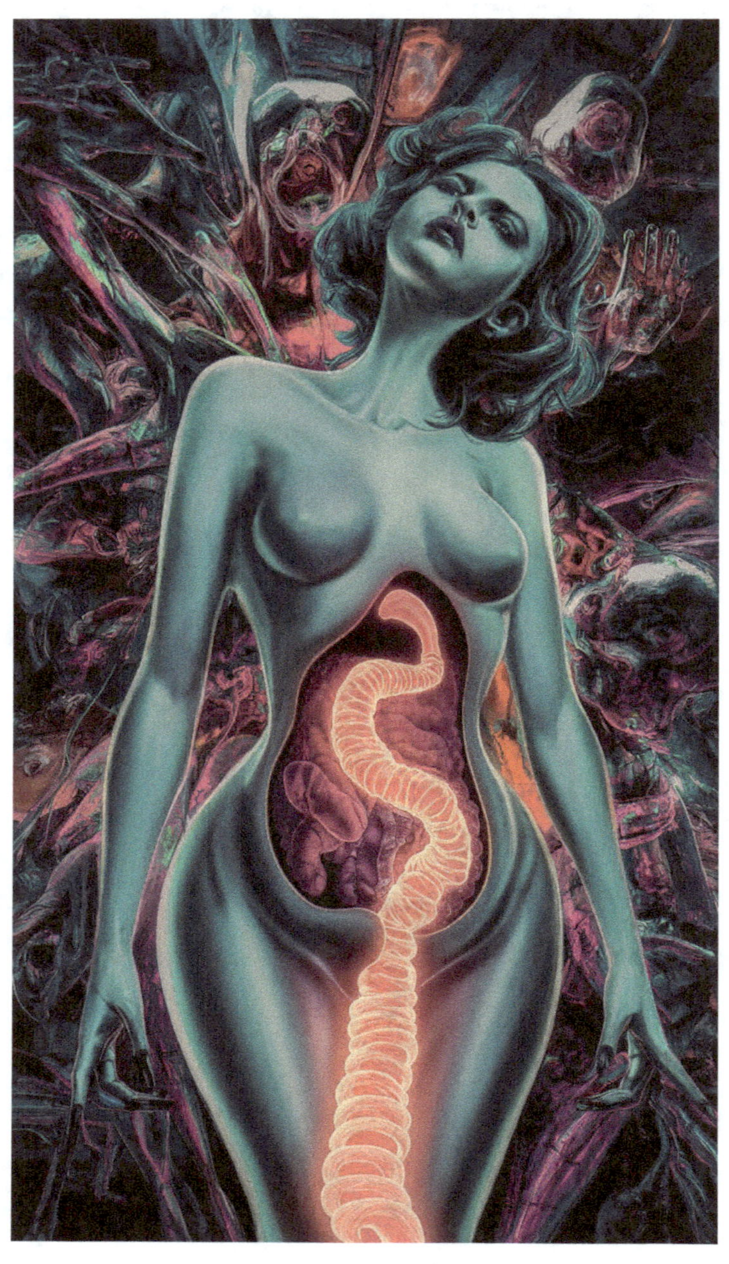

The Host of Beauty

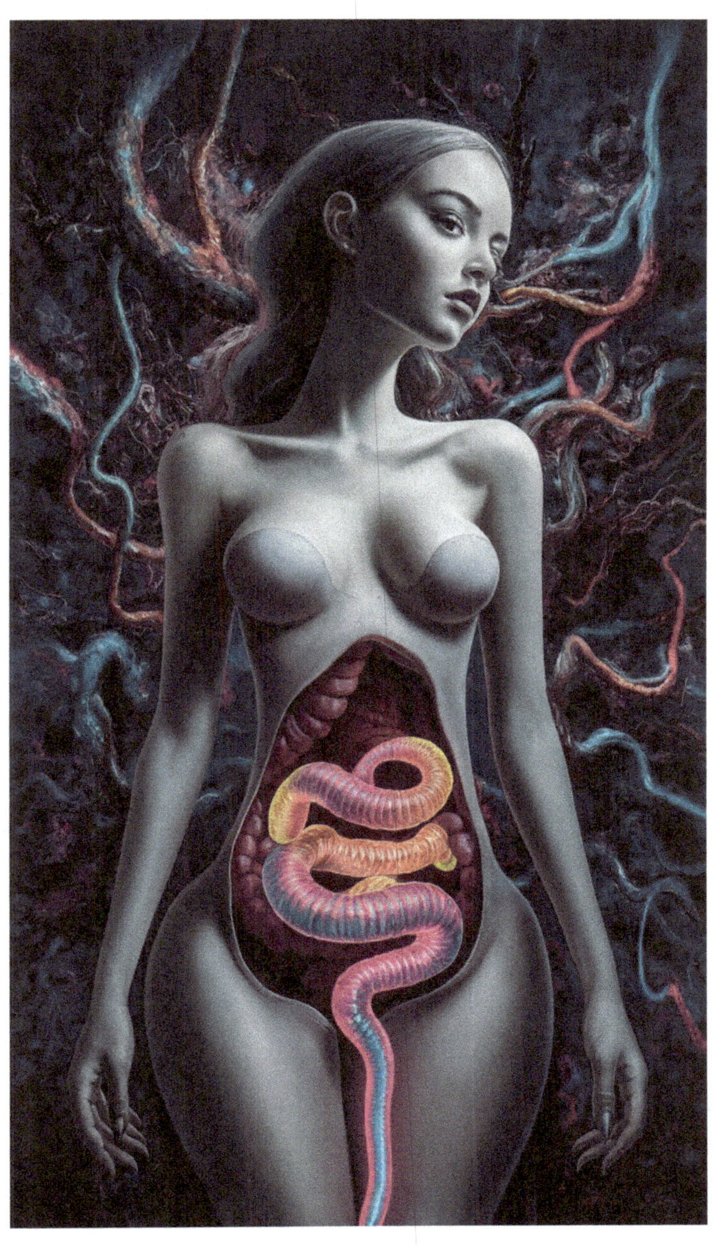

The Parasite Within

The Important of Balanced Approaches

It's important to understand that Ozempic, like any pharmaceutical option, is not a miracle solution for weight loss. While it may help suppress appetite and kickstart weight loss, achieving lasting results requires a more comprehensive approach. This includes balanced nutrition, regular exercise, and healthy lifestyle habits. Relying solely on medication without making these changes is unlikely to lead to sustainable success.

The Pitfalls of Extreme Measures

The growing trend of celebrities using Ozempic for rapid weight loss reflects a broader societal fixation on quick-fix solutions and aesthetic ideals. While these extreme measures may produce visible short-term results, they often come with significant risks and potential consequences for both physical and mental health. It's important for individuals, whether celebrities or not, to prioritize sustainable and balanced approaches to diet and exercise that promote overall well-being, rather than focusing solely on achieving aesthetic goals.

The rise in Ozempic use for weight loss highlights the complex relationship between pharmaceutical innovation, societal pressures, and personal health goals. While it may offer potential as a weight management tool, its off-label use requires careful consideration of both the benefits and risks. In the end, the pursuit of health and well-being should focus on sustainable practices that support long-term physical and mental wellness.

Conspiracy Theories and Dark Secrets

Celebrity culture is often intertwined with conspiracy theories and whispers of dark secrets. Rumors circulate about secret societies and underground networks where the rich and famous engage in mysterious rituals and practices to maintain their youth and vitality. While many of these claims remain unproven, they continue to fuel fascination and intrigue around the endless pursuit of eternal youth.

Unveiling the Mysteries: Secret Societies and the Entertainment Industry

Few topics have captured the collective imagination quite like secret societies. Among the most enigmatic of these groups, the Illuminati and the Freemasons are frequently at the center of conspiracy theories. Cloaked in secrecy and filled with mystique, these clandestine organizations have long been the subject of speculation, with conspiracy theorists attributing to them great influence over various aspects of society, including the entertainment industry.

Central to these conspiracy theories is the belief that members of secret societies participate in elaborate rituals and ceremonies that allegedly grant them extraordinary power, wealth, and even immortality. These rituals, often described as occult practices filled with symbolic and mystical elements, are said to bestow supernatural abilities on participants. According to proponents of these ideas, the ultimate goal of such rituals is to assert control over society and manipulate the course of history itself.

A key component of these conspiracy theories is the alleged influence of secret societies over the entertainment industry. It's suggested that members of these organizations hold powerful roles as executives, producers, and artists, giving them control over media outlets, record labels, and production companies. Through this influence, they are believed to shape cultural narratives and sway public opinion, all while promoting their own agenda and advancing their interests behind the scenes.

Conspiracy theorists often highlight symbolic imagery and references in music videos, films, and television shows as supposed evidence of secret society involvement. From hidden messages in song lyrics to subtle symbolism in album artwork, nearly every aspect of entertainment media is scrutinized for traces of occult influence. These interpretations strengthen the belief that the entertainment industry is a tool for spreading the ideologies of secret societies to the general public, fueling the idea that these groups are using media to shape cultural and societal norms.

It's important to approach these conspiracy theories with a critical perspective. While they may intrigue and entertain, they often lack solid evidence to support their claims. The idea that secret societies control the entertainment industry is largely speculative, based more on conjecture than on verifiable facts. Without concrete proof, these theories remain captivating stories rather than established truths.

Additionally, many of the rituals and ceremonies attributed to secret societies are rooted more in myth and legend than in documented fact. In reality, the entertainment industry is a complex ecosystem shaped by various influences, including market dynamics, artistic expression, and cultural trends. While powerful individuals and organizations certainly play a role in shaping the industry, attributing its operations solely to the influence of secret societies oversimplifies the situation and overlooks the creative agency and diverse factors that drive the entertainment world.

Unveiling the Dark Mysteries of Hollywood

Rumors persist about a hidden world where fame and fortune are said to come with a chilling price. The conspiracy theory surrounding blood sacrifices and occult rituals among celebrities touches on a darker side of the entertainment industry's allure. In this story, the quest for power and immortality collides with the shadowy depths of human desire.

At first glance, these claims might seem far-fetched, easily dismissed as products of overactive imaginations or sensationalist media. But when examined more closely, a darker narrative begins to take shape—a narrative built on speculation, media hype, and society's insatiable curiosity about the lives of the rich and famous. The allure of these stories lies not only in their shocking nature but also in the fascination with the hidden world of celebrity.

A key element of this conspiracy theory is the notion that, behind the closed doors of Hollywood's elite, celebrities participate in secretive, dark rituals—sacrificing blood and soul in pursuit of success, fame, and eternal youth. These clandestine gatherings, veiled in mystery and hidden from public view, are believed to be the backdrop for sinister pacts with dark forces, where the line between reality and myth fades into obscurity.

Rumors of celebrities engaging in strange ceremonies —ranging from animal sacrifices to dark magic rituals— frequently circulate within conspiracy communities and tabloid media, casting an eerie shadow over Hollywood's glamorous image. Behind the glittering facade of fame, a darker narrative takes shape, where the pursuit of worldly desires is believed to come at a sinister cost to the soul. These stories fuel a fascination with the idea of an underworld lurking just beyond the spotlight, one where fame and fortune demand a hidden price.

Names like Beyoncé, Jay-Z, and Lady Gaga often surface in conspiracy circles as being linked to these rumored clandestine practices. Although no concrete evidence exists to support such claims, their high-profile status in the entertainment industry makes them frequent subjects of speculation and scrutiny. Whether these rumors are grounded in reality or simply a reflection of the public's fascination with the darker aspects of celebrity life is left open to interpretation. The persistent buzz around these figures highlights the enduring allure of such conspiracy theories in the realm of fame.

The pursuit of eternal youth takes many forms, from the cosmetic procedures of Beverly Hills to the murky corners of conspiracy theories. When we look beyond the surface of celebrity culture, we see a world where vanity and insecurity intertwine, pushing individuals to take drastic measures in their quest for the elusive fountain of youth. Beneath the glitz and glamour, however, lies the hidden cost of these endeavors— masked by the facade of perfection and the irresistible allure of everlasting beauty.

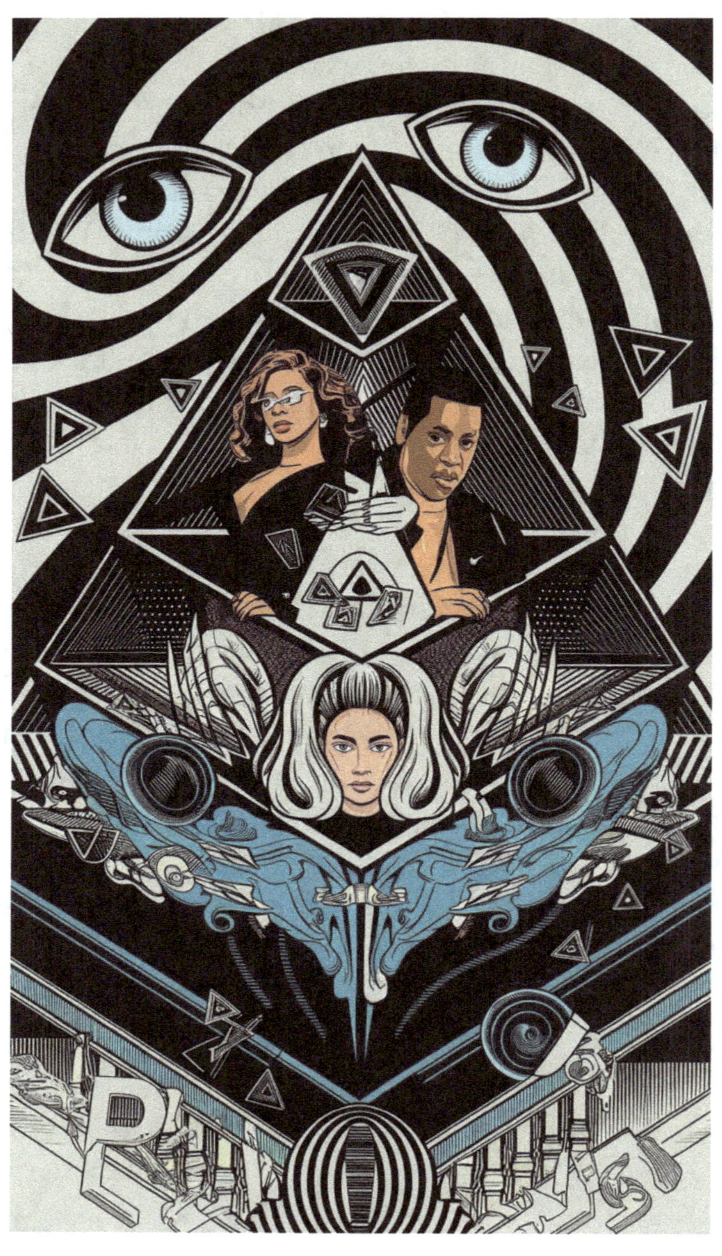

The Triangle of Influence: Beyonce, Jay Z, and Lady Gaga

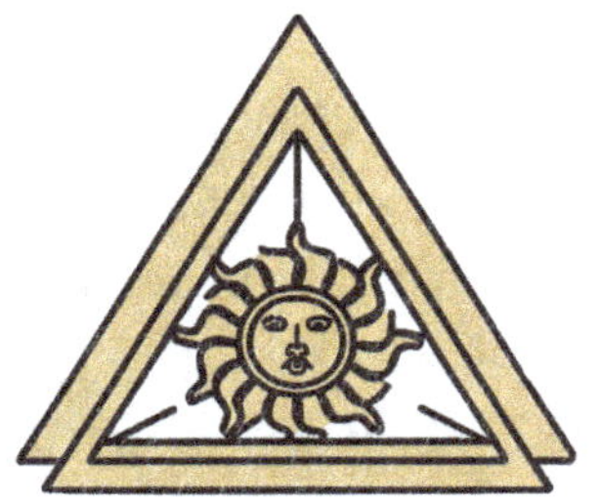

Chapter 2: The Hidden Costs of Perfection

Chasing youth is like chasing the horizon; you never quite reach it, but you miss the beauty of where you are.

Celebrities, caught in the pursuit of eternal youth and physical perfection, often find themselves trapped in a web of pressures, expectations, and sacrifices. While the temptation to maintain a flawless appearance may appear irresistible from the outside, the reality behind the glamorous facade reveals a much darker truth—a world consumed by obsession, insecurity, and an unending quest for impossible standards.

The Pressure to Conform

The pressure to meet society's beauty standards is a widespread issue, impacting individuals in many industries, particularly in entertainment. Celebrities, in particular, are often under intense scrutiny for their appearance, held to nearly impossible standards of beauty and perfection. This pressure comes from many directions, including relentless media attention and harsh criticism from both fans hind industry insiders, creating a challenging environment for those in the spotlight.

For many celebrities, the pressure to fit into narrow beauty standards starts early in their careers and can have profound psychological and emotional effects. The constant focus on physical appearance often leads to body image issues, low self-esteem, and even struggles with mental health. This relentless emphasis on looks creates a challenging environment that can be difficult to navigate, both personally and professionally.

Beyond physical appearance, the pressure to conform also affects other aspects of a celebrity's life, including their behavior, lifestyle choices, and public image. Celebrities often feel the need to maintain a certain persona that fits societal expectations, even when it doesn't align with who they truly are. This can create a sense of inauthenticity, leaving them feeling trapped in a cycle of constantly performing for the public rather than living as their genuine selves.

Actress Megan Fox's recent remarks offer a powerful example of the challenges faced by women, particularly new mothers, in Hollywood. The *Transformers* star openly discussed the unrealistic expectations placed on working mothers, sharing her own struggles to meet the industry's strict beauty standards shortly after giving birth. Fox's candidness sheds light on the deep-rooted patriarchal norms in Hollywood, where women are expected to quickly return to their pre-pregnancy bodies and resume their careers with little support or understanding. Her experience underscores the internal conflict many women face, balancing societal pressures with the need to prioritize their health and the well-being of their newborns. By speaking out, Fox highlights the need for more empathy and flexibility in an industry that often places appearance above the overall needs of women and their families.

The pressure to conform to rigid beauty standards is a complicated issue that affects both celebrities and everyday individuals. It highlights the need to challenge societal expectations, encourage diversity and inclusivity, and cultivate a culture of acceptance and self-love. By embracing these values, we can move toward a more positive and inclusive definition of beauty that celebrates individuality rather than forcing everyone to fit into a narrow mold.

Obsession and Compulsion

The pursuit of physical perfection can easily spiral into an overwhelming obsession, dominating the lives of those entangled in its grasp. Celebrities, in particular, may find themselves consumed by the need to constantly track calories, meticulously monitor their bodies, and strive for an unattainable ideal. This relentless focus on perfection often comes at a steep cost, leading to the sacrifice of their health, happiness, and even mental well-being as they chase the ever-elusive image of flawlessness.

The pursuit of physical perfection can quickly evolve into an all-encompassing obsession, trapping individuals in a cycle of constant focus and compulsion. For many celebrities, what begins as a desire for an ideal body often becomes a singular, dominating force that influences every aspect of their lives. This obsession typically reveals itself through meticulous behaviors and an unrelenting drive to meet an impossible standard of perfection, overshadowing other priorities and well-being.

Calorie counting can quickly escalate from a simple tool for managing dietary intake to a rigid routine governed by strict numerical goals. Every bite of food is meticulously weighed, measured, and logged, with any deviation from the plan often leading to intense guilt and self-criticism. This relentless quest for achieving a certain body weight or appearance can foster unhealthy behaviors, including extreme dieting, disordered eating habits, and, in severe cases, the development of eating disorders such as anorexia nervosa or bulimia.

In addition to strict dieting, celebrities can often find themselves stuck in a cycle of obsessive self-monitoring, constantly examining their bodies for perceived flaws or imperfections. What might start as a simple desire for self-improvement can quickly spiral into an unending pursuit of physical flawlessness. This obsession manifests through frequent body checking, mirror gazing, and endless comparisons to the unrealistic beauty ideals that media and society promote. This idea is portrayed greatly in the recent 2024 film, *The Substance* with Demi Moore where Demi Moore's character spirals out of control once she gets her hands on a miraculous "substance" that creates a more "perfect" and younger version of herself. She becomes addicted to this younger version of herself ultimately leading to her demise.

Driven by the desire to meet unattainable beauty ideals, celebrities often take drastic steps, from undergoing multiple cosmetic surgeries to following intense workout routines, or even turning to dangerous substances or supplements to achieve their ideal look. The constant pressure to conform to these unrealistic standards can take a serious toll on their mental and emotional health, often resulting in increased levels of anxiety, depression, and even body dysmorphia.

The relentless pursuit of physical perfection often takes a significant toll on celebrities, stripping away their health, happiness, and self-esteem. While the allure of external praise and the desire to embody an idealized image may seem tempting, the reality is that striving for perfection frequently leads to a sense of emptiness. This unattainable goal traps individuals in a cycle of dissatisfaction, where no achievement feels good enough, leaving them vulnerable to both physical and emotional harm.

Judy Garland's story stands as a powerful reminder of the dangers that come with Hollywood's relentless pressure for physical perfection. Thrust into fame at just sixteen, Garland quickly found herself under the microscope of studio executives who were determined to shape her into the ideal image of feminine beauty. Despite her incredible talent and undeniable charisma, her career was affected by the overwhelming pressure to meet impossible standards of thinness and glamour. In her memoirs and interviews, Garland openly spoke about the extreme demands placed on her to lose weight and stick to rigid diet plans, which deeply impacted both her physical health and emotional well-being.

Garland's struggles with fame and body image were intensified by a deeper issue: addiction. Caught in a whirlwind created by the demands of the studio system, she was introduced to amphetamines and other prescription drugs at a young age. These pills, handed to her under the guise of suppressing her appetite and boosting her energy, were meant to keep her going through grueling filming schedules. What began as a way to cope with the relentless pace of Hollywood soon evolved into something far more damaging. The dependency on these substances took hold, tightening its grip as her reliance on them grew, ultimately leading her into a cycle of addiction. This spiral only magnified her battles with mental health and self-worth, pulling her deeper into a dangerous path paved by those who profited from her success.

The studio's indifferent approach to Judy Garland's well-being, along with the widespread normalization of substance use in Hollywood, played a significant role in her downward spiral. Instead of addressing the deeper issues that fueled her self-destructive behavior, executives prioritized the bottom line, ignoring the warning signs of her growing dependency. In this toxic environment, Garland was left vulnerable, trapped in a cycle of addiction with little support to help her escape its clutches. As her struggles intensified, the industry continued to profit from her talent while turning a blind eye to the suffering it perpetuated.

Judy Garland's heartbreaking end serves as a powerful reminder of the darker side of Hollywood's allure and the devastating effects of exploitation and neglect. Her battles with body image, addiction, and mental health highlight the heavy price paid by those in an industry that often prioritizes physical appearance over human well-being. Garland's immense talent, overshadowed by these struggles, was ultimately lost far too soon, leaving behind a legacy that reflects both her brilliance and the tragic cost of the pressures she faced.

Many celebrities, despite their fame and luxury, struggle with profound insecurities and self-doubt. Constantly being compared to their peers and facing relentless pressure to maintain a youthful image can take a toll on their self-esteem, often eroding their sense of self-worth. This leaves them trapped in a cycle of dissatisfaction and self-loathing, despite the outward appearance of success and glamour.

It's tempting to believe that celebrities live effortlessly glamorous lives, free from the burdens of insecurity or self-doubt. However, behind the glittering façade of red carpet appearances and glossy magazine covers, there's a more complicated reality. Despite their outward success and seemingly flawless lives, many celebrities struggle with deep feelings of inadequacy and self-doubt, fueled by the constant scrutiny and high expectations that come with life in the entertainment industry.

A quick glance at the headlines reveals how deeply the culture of comparison and judgment runs in Hollywood. Tabloids and social media platforms often become battlegrounds for relentless criticism and scrutiny. Celebrities face constant evaluation—not only from the media and fans but also from their peers within the industry. The immense pressure to meet narrow beauty standards and maintain a flawless appearance can take a significant toll on their self-esteem, fostering feelings of insecurity and inadequacy.

Even the most accomplished and celebrated stars are not exempt from grappling with insecurities. A prime example is Academy Award-winning actress Jennifer Lawrence, who has openly discussed her struggles with body image and self-confidence amid Hollywood's unrealistic beauty standards. In various interviews, Lawrence has shared moments where she felt immense pressure to meet impossible ideals of thinness and perfection, leading her to question her own worth as both an actress and a woman. These experiences highlight the profound impact that the entertainment industry's standards can have on even the most successful figures.

Likewise, pop superstar Lady Gaga has been open about her struggles with self-doubt and insecurity, despite her incredible rise to fame and critical success. In her documentary *Gaga: Five Foot Two*, she reveals her vulnerabilities, giving viewers a glimpse into the emotional turmoil that accompanies life in the spotlight. Gaga's honest reflections remind us that even the most iconic and accomplished figures in the entertainment world are not immune to feelings of inadequacy and self-doubt, offering a powerful reminder of the personal battles many face behind the scenes.

The constant pressure to preserve a youthful appearance only amplifies feelings of insecurity and doubt among celebrities, who are continuously exposed to idealized images of perfection. Whether through age-defying cosmetic treatments or airbrushed magazine covers, the underlying message is unmistakable: youth equals beauty, and anything else falls short. This harmful narrative fuels a cycle of self-criticism and dissatisfaction, trapping many stars in an endless pursuit of validation and acceptance, often leaving them feeling inadequate and undeserving.

Insecurity and self-doubt aren't just abstract notions—they're real challenges that profoundly affect the lives of many celebrities. Despite their wealth and public admiration, numerous stars struggle with overwhelming feelings of inadequacy and worthlessness, unable to escape the relentless pressures of the entertainment world. It serves as a stark reminder that behind the fame and glamour lies a reality filled with vulnerability, where even the most celebrated figures aren't immune to the weight of self-doubt.

Body Dysmorphia and Dysmorphic Disorder

For some individuals, the relentless chase for physical perfection can spiral into a serious mental health condition known as body dysmorphic disorder (BDD). This disorder is marked by an obsessive focus on perceived flaws or imperfections in one's appearance, often minor or even imagined. BDD can wreak havoc on a person's life, leading to severe consequences such as social withdrawal, deep depression, and in extreme cases, self-harm or suicidal thoughts.

Actress Megan Fox, renowned for her striking appearance and magnetic presence on screen, has been open about her struggles with Body Dysmorphic Disorder (BDD), shedding light on the hidden challenges that often accompany fame and beauty. In several heartfelt interviews, Fox has discussed the deep-seated insecurities and self-doubt that have followed her throughout her career, revealing that, despite her outward success, the pressure to maintain a perfect image has taken a significant toll on her mental well-being.

For Fox, the constant scrutiny of her looks and the unrealistic beauty standards promoted by the entertainment world had a serious impact on her mental well-being. She found herself obsessively focusing on every perceived flaw and feeling immense pressure to fit into society's narrow definition of beauty. This pressure led her into a damaging cycle of self-criticism and dissatisfaction, as she struggled to meet expectations that felt impossible to achieve.

Throughout her journey to confront and overcome BDD, Fox has become a strong advocate for self-acceptance and body positivity. She's used her platform to push back against the toxic beauty standards so prevalent in Hollywood. By openly sharing her personal struggles with honesty and vulnerability, Fox has inspired many of her fans to embrace their imperfections and celebrate their unique qualities. In doing so, she has helped shift the focus away from superficial ideals, encouraging others to recognize the true beauty that lies within.

The emergence of social media has intensified the spread of BDD among celebrities, with platforms like Instagram, TikTok and Twitter amplifying the culture of comparison and perfectionism. The constant need to project a flawless image under endless scrutiny can drive vulnerable individuals deeper into feelings of inadequacy. This pressure often fuels a destructive cycle of self-criticism and harmful behaviors, making it increasingly difficult for those affected to break free from the weight of unrealistic beauty standards.

In the high-pressure environment of show business, where physical appearance often dictates success, body dysmorphic disorder casts a heavy shadow over the lives of many celebrities. While the glamour of fame and fortune may bring fleeting moments of validation, they offer little comfort to those struggling with BDD. For these individuals, every glance in the mirror reflects a distorted perception of self-worth, creating a cycle of insecurity and self-criticism that is difficult to escape.

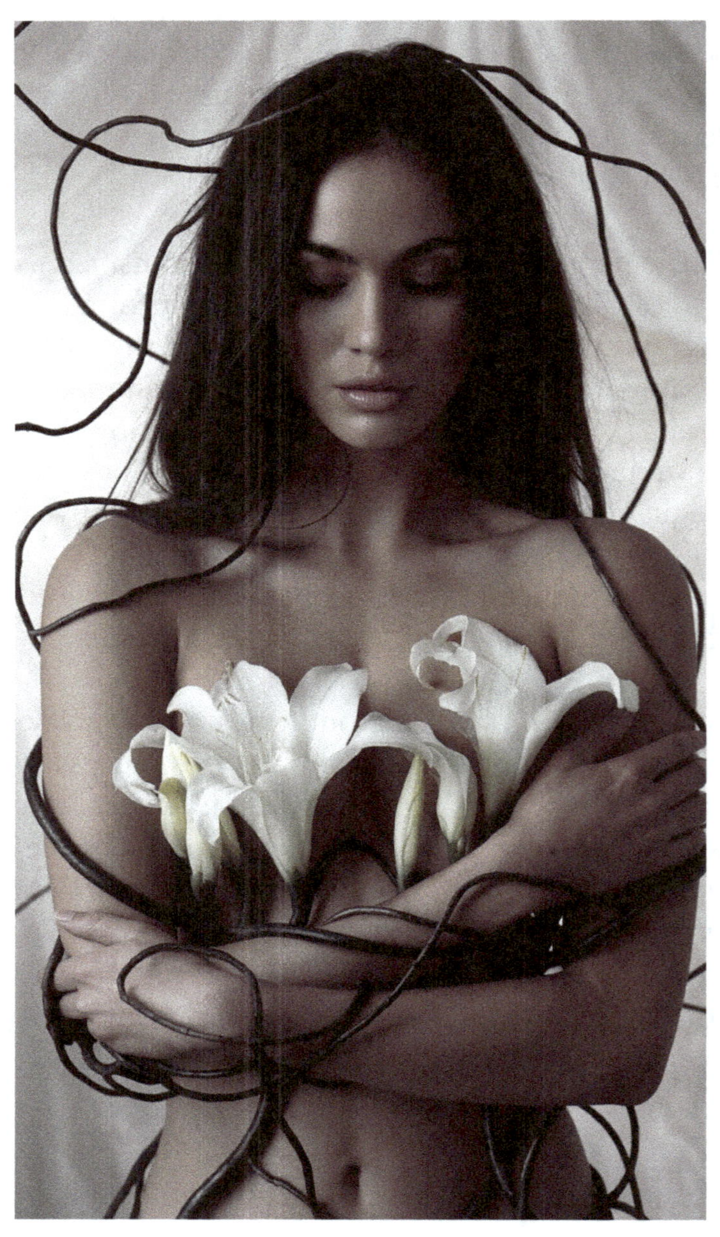

Megan Fox: Beauty Entwined

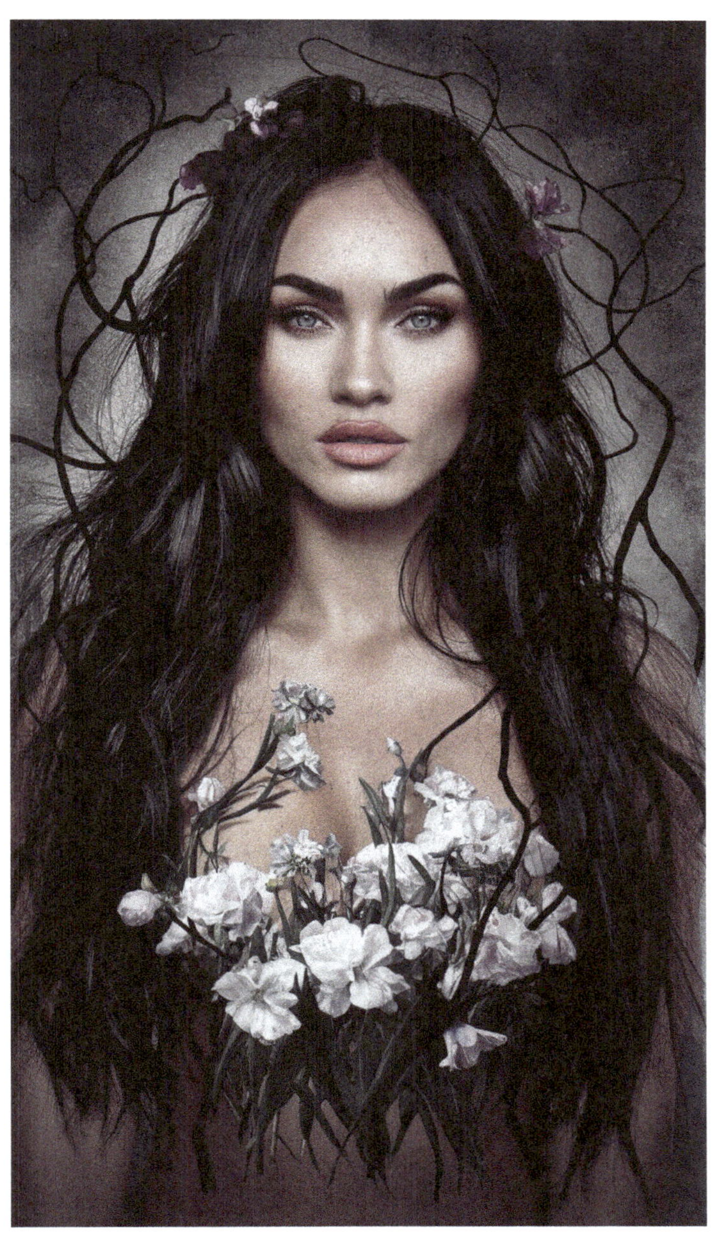

The Naked Truth with Megan Fox

The pursuit of physical perfection takes a significant toll on celebrities' personal lives, relationships, and overall well-being. The unrelenting demands of fame often leave little room for self-care or reflection, leading to burnout, exhaustion, and emotional distress.

Celebrities like Selena Gomez and Demi Lovato have openly discussed the impact fame has had on their mental health, revealing the often-hidden struggles within the entertainment industry. Gomez, in particular, has been transparent about her battles with anxiety and depression, pointing to the immense pressure of fame and the relentless media scrutiny as significant contributors to her emotional challenges. Their honesty has helped to expose the darker side of stardom, where constant public attention can take a serious toll on well-being.

Demi Lovato has also been open about her struggles with addiction, eating disorders, and self-harm, shedding light on how the pressures of fame can deeply affect mental health. Both Lovato and Selena Gomez's experiences reveal the deep loneliness, isolation, and disillusionment that often come with living in the spotlight, despite the outward appearances of success and glamour. Their stories serve as powerful reminders that life in the public eye can take a heavy toll on emotional well-being, regardless of how perfect things may seem on the surface.

When the spotlight dims and the cameras stop flashing, celebrities are left to face the difficult truths that come with fame—the toll it takes on their mental and emotional health, the sacrifices they make in their personal lives, and the unrelenting pressure to uphold an image of perfection. In their pursuit of physical perfection, many find themselves caught in a cycle of loneliness, isolation, and disappointment, longing for genuine connection and authenticity amidst the surface-level nature of celebrity culture.

The Illusion of Perfection

With the rise of social media and advanced photo editing tools, the distinction between authenticity and illusion becomes increasingly harder to define. Celebrities, facing constant pressure to appear flawless, often turn to extreme diets, cosmetic surgeries, or digital alterations to uphold a picture-perfect image. This relentless drive for perfection fuels unattainable beauty standards, causing many to grapple with feelings of inadequacy and unworthiness.

Social media platforms like Instagram, with their perfectly curated and filtered images, play a significant role in promoting unrealistic beauty standards. Celebrities often feel pressured to appear flawless and meticulously groomed at all times, anxious about the fallout from even the slightest imperfection. This constant chase for perfection takes a toll on their mental and physical health, while also reinforcing beauty ideals that are virtually impossible for the average person to attain.

The increasing use of digital manipulation tools has made it even easier for celebrities to alter their appearances in photos and videos, blurring the line between reality and fantasy. With just a few clicks, wrinkles are smoothed, features are enhanced, and an idealized version of beauty is created—one that is impossible to achieve without the help of technology. This manufactured image of perfection can have a damaging effect, especially on young, impressionable fans, who may internalize these unrealistic standards and struggle with feelings of inadequacy when they don't measure up.

Many celebrities find themselves trapped by the pressure to maintain a flawless image, constantly scrutinized by fans, the media, and industry insiders. In a world where appearance often defines success, the demand to align with conventional beauty standards can feel overwhelming. This constant pressure leads some stars to take extreme measures in their efforts to meet societal expectations, reinforcing the idea that image is everything in the entertainment industry.

Few families in popular culture have wielded as much influence as the Kardashians, whose omnipresence on social media has significantly shaped beauty standards and cultural norms. However, their frequent use of digital alterations in their photos has sparked widespread criticism, with accusations of excessive photoshopping and retouching becoming a common theme. This practice has far-reaching effects, especially on impressionable young girls who may come to see these edited images as the ultimate standard of perfection.

The flood of heavily edited photos across social media distorts perceptions of reality, fostering unattainable expectations and leaving many feeling inadequate for not achieving the same level of flawlessness. As a result, the Kardashian family's reliance on editing tools not only reinforces unrealistic beauty standards but also fuels the toxic culture of comparison and self-doubt prevalent on social platforms. It highlights the critical need to encourage authenticity and transparency in celebrity representation, challenging the overwhelming influence of digitally altered images and pushing for a more inclusive and realistic definition of beauty.

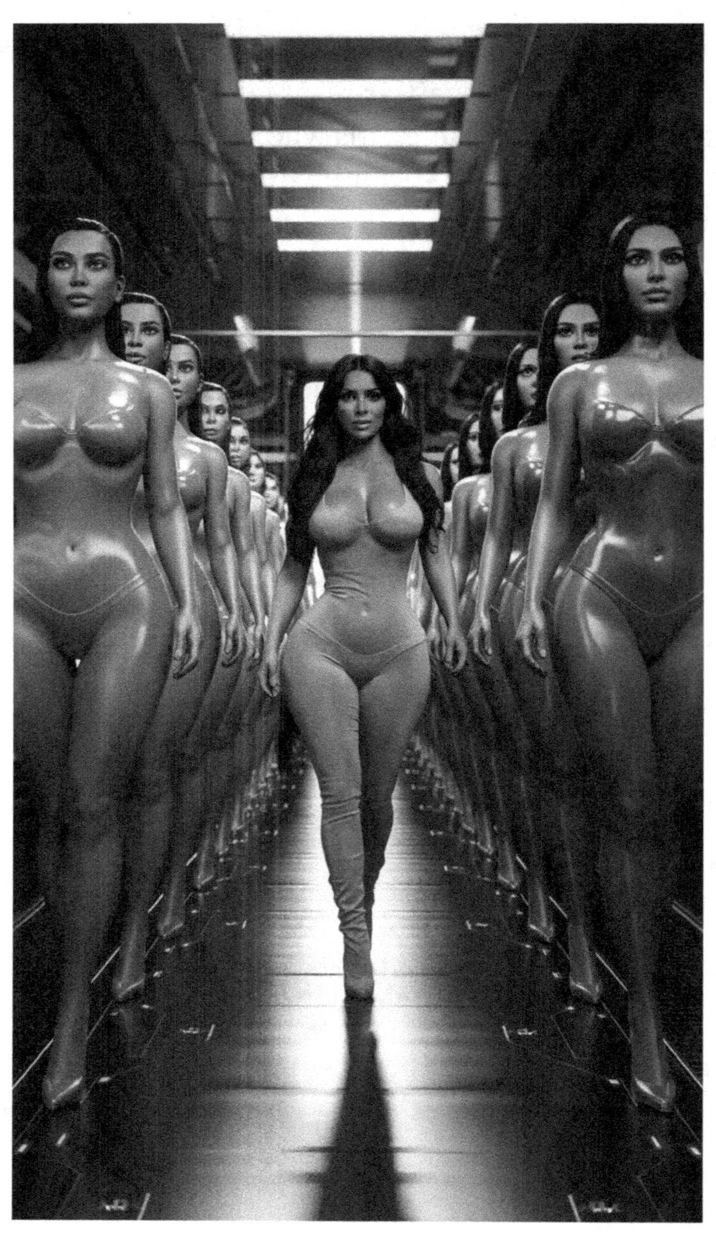

Kim Kardashian: The Plastic Illusion

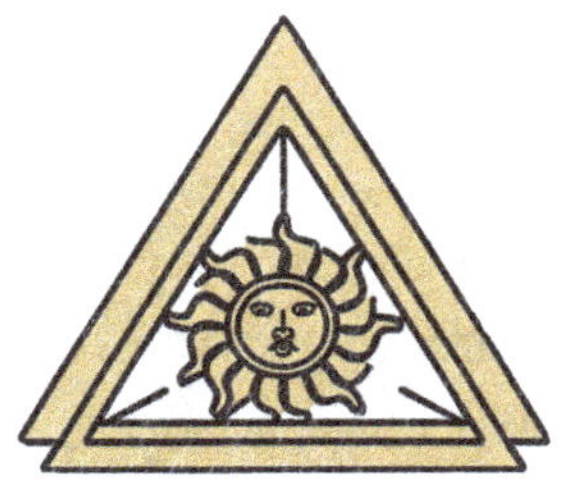

Chapter 3: Wild and Bizarre Methods of Anti-Aging Throughout History

The fountain of youth is not a place, but a myth born of desperation—a reflection of humanity's refusal to accept time's truth.

Throughout history, the desire for eternal youth has captivated the elite, leading them to explore unconventional, and sometimes bizarre, methods in their quest to defy aging. From ancient empires to medieval and Renaissance courts, there are countless stories of people searching for mystical elixirs, magical potions, and age-defying rituals that promised to stop or even reverse the natural aging process.

These age-defying practices were often rooted in superstition, mysticism, and folklore, reflecting the beliefs and cultural norms of their time. In ancient civilizations like Egypt and China, alchemists sought to transform base metals into gold and uncover the elusive elixir of life, believing these substances held the secret to immortality. Similarly, during the Middle Ages, European nobility turned to alchemy, astrology, and herbal remedies in their pursuit of eternal youth, often with questionable outcomes. The Renaissance brought renewed interest in longevity, with people experimenting with various potions, tonics, and herbal remedies in the hope of maintaining their youth and vitality. While many of these practices may seem fantastical or even absurd today, they reveal the timeless human desire to defy aging and escape mortality.

Veins of Vitality: Unraveling the Ancient Mysteries of Bloodletting

Throughout medical history, few practices have sparked as much curiosity and puzzlement as bloodletting. Bloodletting was a prominent practice that spanned from the ancient temples of Mesopotamia to the healing chambers of Egypt. It was deeply rooted in the medical theory of humoralism, which claimed that the body's health depended on the balance of four key fluids, or humors. Practitioners believed that by removing excess blood, they could restore this balance, bringing the body's humors into harmony and ultimately improving a patient's vitality and well-being. This method became a foundational element of ancient medical treatments, reflecting the long-held belief that blood held the key to healing and rejuvenation.

The Ritual Unveiled

Bloodletting was far from a straightforward procedure—it was a delicate and ritualistic exchange between healer and patient, with health often teetering on the edge. Practitioners used a variety of techniques, from venesection, where veins were deliberately cut to release blood, to the use of leeches, those slippery creatures once believed to possess unique healing properties. Each approach came with its own set of risks and potential benefits, promising either restoration of vitality or the threat of harm, depending on the skill of the healer and the patient's response.

The Illusion of Rejuvenation

For centuries, bloodletting captivated both healers and patients, casting a spell over the medical world. Esteemed figures like Hippocrates and Galen championed the practice, praising its supposed ability to cure countless ailments. Its reputation as a universal remedy became deeply ingrained in the fabric of ancient medicine. However, beneath the surface of these revered endorsements lay a harsh reality—what seemed like rejuvenation was often a dangerous illusion. Instead of restoring health, bloodletting frequently left patients weaker, their energy drained along with the blood they so desperately needed.

The Tragic End of a Leader: George Washington's Fatal Encounter with Bloodletting

Among the most tragic and illustrative moments of outdated medical practices is the death of George Washington, the esteemed first President of the United States. His passing in December 1799 serves as a powerful reminder of the dangers that lurked within the once widely-accepted practice of bloodletting.

In the cold winter of 1799, 67-year-old George Washington found himself stricken with a severe sore throat that left him gravely ill. Seeking relief, he turned to his trusted physicians, Dr. James Craik and Dr. Gustavus Brown.

The Fateful Intervention

Following the medical practices of the time, Washington's doctors began a series of bloodletting sessions, believing it would help balance his bodily humors and relieve his symptoms. Over the span of several hours, they drew a substantial amount of blood from the ailing president in a determined effort to improve his condition. Despite their best intentions, Washington's health continued to decline at an alarming rate, with each procedure offering no reprieve from his worsening state.

On the evening of December 14, 1799, George Washington took his final breath, leaving the young nation in a state of deep mourning. The loss of such a revered leader and founding father sent shockwaves throughout the country. While the exact nature of Washington's illness remains debated by historians and medical professionals, many believe the extensive bloodletting he endured likely played a significant role in hastening his death.

The Legacy of Bloodletting

Despite its dangers and questionable effectiveness, bloodletting remained a cornerstone of medical practice well into the 19th century. Its story is woven into the fabric of history, symbolizing humanity's relentless pursuit of health and vitality. While modern medicine has relegated bloodletting to the past, its legacy still lingers—a reminder of the fascinating and often mysterious path that has shaped our understanding of healing through the ages.

The Alchemist's Quest: Unraveling the Mysteries of Immortality

In the shadowy halls of medieval castles and the lavish rooms of Renaissance courts, an air of mystery seemed to hang in the atmosphere—whispers of hidden knowledge and untold secrets. At the center of this fascination was the ancient practice of alchemy, a captivating and mysterious pursuit that enthralled both scholars and the elite. Alchemy promised transformation, the discovery of profound truths, and the allure of turning ordinary substances into extraordinary ones.

The Promise of Immortality

Throughout the medieval and Renaissance eras, alchemy emerged as a beacon of hope in an unpredictable world. At the heart of this pursuit was the tantalizing myth of the philosopher's stone—a fabled substance thought to possess the power of transmutation and the key to eternal life. Alchemists, including some of the wealthiest and most influential figures of their time, devoted their lives to seeking this elusive elixir. They conducted intricate experiments and scoured ancient texts, all in the hopes of uncovering the hidden formulas that would unlock the secrets of immortality.

The Alchemist's Patronage

Many influential figures across the ages were drawn to the mysteries of alchemy, eager to unlock its secrets and harness its potential power. From royalty and nobility to scholars and visionaries, alchemy's patrons invested heavily in their quest for enlightenment. Notable individuals like Holy Roman Emperor Rudolf II and King James IV of Scotland stood among those who sponsored alchemists, providing them with laboratories, equipment, and resources to fuel their research. Behind the scenes, away from prying eyes, these alchemists toiled tirelessly, conducting experiments and exploring the unknown in their relentless pursuit of the philosopher's stone.

Alchemy: A Journey of the Soul

Alchemy was more than just a pursuit of material wealth or power—it was a profound spiritual and philosophical journey aimed at unlocking the mysteries of the universe. Alchemists believed that transmuting base metals into noble ones symbolized the transformation of the soul on its path to enlightenment. Their experiments went beyond chemistry, encompassing everything from the distillation of potions and elixirs to studying astrological influences and interpreting mystical symbols. Each endeavor, they believed, brought them closer to the ultimate truth they sought to uncover.

The Legacy of Alchemy

Though alchemy's ambitions were grand and its influence profound, it ultimately fell short of delivering on its promises. The philosopher's stone remained an unattainable goal, and many alchemists devoted their lives to the pursuit without ever finding success. Still, alchemy's legacy endures as a symbol of humanity's relentless quest for knowledge, understanding, and the secrets of immortality. The alchemist's journey is etched into history—a reflection of the human spirit's unyielding determination, forever striving toward the unattainable elixir of life.

Elixir of Immortality: The Mystique of Exotic Remedies

Throughout history, whispered rumors have spoken of elites indulging in exotic concoctions, driven by their desire for longevity and vitality. These individuals sought out substances believed to possess mystical properties—from powdered gemstones to rare herbs and parts of exotic animals. These elusive elixirs were thought to unlock the secrets of eternal youth and spiritual enlightenment. While the true effectiveness of these practices remains a mystery, the fascination with these exotic remedies endures, threading a tale of intrigue through the corridors of time.

The Mystical Power of Gemstones

Among the most sought-after substances were powdered gemstones, prized for their radiant colors and believed to embody the earth's elemental energies. In ancient civilizations such as Egypt and Mesopotamia, elites would either consume or apply these powdered gems, convinced that they could harness the unique properties of each stone. From the fiery intensity of rubies to the calming essence of sapphires, every gemstone was revered for its supposed power to grant strength, vitality, and spiritual enlightenment to those fortunate enough to use them.

Botanical Wonders from Distant Lands

In a similar vein, rare herbs and botanicals from far-off lands captivated those in search of longevity and vitality. From the misty peaks of the Orient to the sun-soaked valleys of the New World, exotic plants were treasured for both their medicinal qualities and mystical allure. Ginseng, a cornerstone of traditional Chinese medicine, was revered for its rejuvenating properties and reputed ability to enhance vitality and extend life.

The elixirs crafted from these botanical marvels promised to reveal the secrets of eternal youth, enticing the elite into a world brimming with enchantment and boundless possibilities.

The Mystique of Exotic Animal Parts

Exotic animal parts also played a significant role in the pursuit of rejuvenation, revered for their potent and rare qualities believed to bestow strength, vitality, and longevity upon those who consumed them. From the powerful tiger to the elusive rhinoceros, certain animal organs or extracts were thought to hold the essence of life's resilience and vigor. Tiger bones, for instance, were once believed to transfer the tiger's formidable strength and ferocity to the person consuming it, while rhinoceros horn was famed for its alleged aphrodisiac properties and ability to promote longevity. These prized substances became highly sought after among the elite, embodying a deep-seated belief in the transformative power of nature's wild creatures.

The Perilous Pursuit of Immortality: Mercury Ingestion in History

Throughout history, a perilous chapter unfolds in the quest for eternal youth—a chapter marked by danger and misguided ambition. Desperation drove some of the most prominent figures, including royalty and nobility, to ingest mercury in a misguided attempt to extend their lives. Despite the well-known risks of mercury poisoning, these individuals placed their faith in the supposed mystical properties of this toxic substance, illustrating the extreme lengths to which people would go in their relentless pursuit of immortality.

The Temptation of Mercury

The belief in ingesting mercury as a path to longevity or immortality dates back to ancient civilizations, where alchemists and healers tirelessly searched for the secrets of eternal life. Mercury, with its liquid form and hypnotic shimmer, carried an aura of mystery that intrigued those who placed faith in the transformative powers of alchemy. Many believed that by consuming mercury, they could purify the body, restore balance to the humors, and achieve a state of everlasting youth and vitality.

The Tragic Consequences

Even without scientific backing, the appeal of mercury endured among the elite throughout history. Desperate to preserve their youth and fend off the signs of aging, some individuals turned to mercury ingestion as a final, misguided solution. The results, however, were disastrous. Mercury is incredibly toxic to the human body, and consuming it led to severe health complications, including damage to the nervous system, kidneys, and digestive organs. Prolonged exposure often resulted in crippling symptoms, organ failure, and in many cases, death.

The Disturbing Tapestry of History:

One of the most disturbing elements in the pursuit of eternal youth lies in the chilling accounts—whether disputed or exaggerated—of elites engaging in rituals involving human sacrifice or even cannibalism. Driven by the belief that consuming the flesh or blood of others would grant them power or extend their lives, these individuals ventured into the darkest depths of human depravity. These practices, whether real or imagined, have left a legacy steeped in horror and revulsion, casting a shadow over history's quest for immortality

Gilles de Rais

A figure steeped in infamy is Gilles de Rais, a French nobleman whose life serves as a haunting example of how power and privilege can spiral into darkness. Known for his bravery as a military leader and his role as a trusted companion to Joan of Arc, de Rais's path took a horrifying twist. He faced shocking accusations involving the torture and murder of children, as well as necrophilia. Although historians still debate the true extent of his involvement in these crimes, the story of Gilles de Rais stands as a chilling reminder of the depths of depravity that can exist among the elite.

Elizabeth Bathory

Another infamous figure in history is Elizabeth Bathory, known as the "Blood Countess" of 16th-century Hungary. She was accused of torturing and murdering hundreds of young women, supposedly under the belief that bathing in their blood would keep her youthful and beautiful. Whether these shocking allegations are entirely true or exaggerated remains a topic of debate, but Bathory's name has become a symbol of aristocratic excess and cruelty. Her story still casts a dark shadow over history, illustrating the terrifying extremes of power and vanity.

Ritualistic Sacrifice in Ancient Civilizations

In ancient times, civilizations like the Aztec Empire practiced ritualistic human sacrifice, carried out by priests and the elite as offerings to their gods. While these rituals were mainly driven by religious and cultural beliefs, there are some indications that certain individuals might have viewed these gruesome practices as a way to achieve rejuvenation or extend their lives by consuming human flesh or blood.

Poisoned Elegance: The Deadly Allure of Toxic Cosmetics

Throughout history, the pursuit of beauty by the elite has been intense, with some going to shocking lengths in their quest for everlasting youth and charm. From ancient civilizations to the glamorous courts of

European nobility, people have used cosmetics laced with toxic substances, leaving behind a haunting legacy of vanity and risk. This shows just how powerful the pull of beauty can be, even when it comes at the expense of one's health.

The Ancient Temptation

In ancient Egypt, people aimed to elevate their beauty to almost divine levels by using cosmetics. One of the most notable products they used was kohl eyeliner, which contained lead—a toxic substance that could create a striking, mesmerizing look but came with the risk of lead poisoning and severe health issues. Despite the dangers, both men and women continued to apply kohl to their eyes, unaware of the hidden risks in their beauty rituals.

The Deadly Elegance of Elizabethan Courts

As time moved forward, the Elizabethan era brought a new wave of elegance and sophistication, marked by the widespread use of arsenic-laced cosmetics in the quest for beauty. From royal courts to the lavish homes of the nobility, faces were covered in powders and creams infused with arsenic—a deadly poison that was believed to create a flawless, pale complexion symbolizing aristocratic grace. Even Queen Elizabeth I was drawn to the dangerous charm of arsenic, using it as part of her relentless pursuit of beauty, despite the risks it posed.

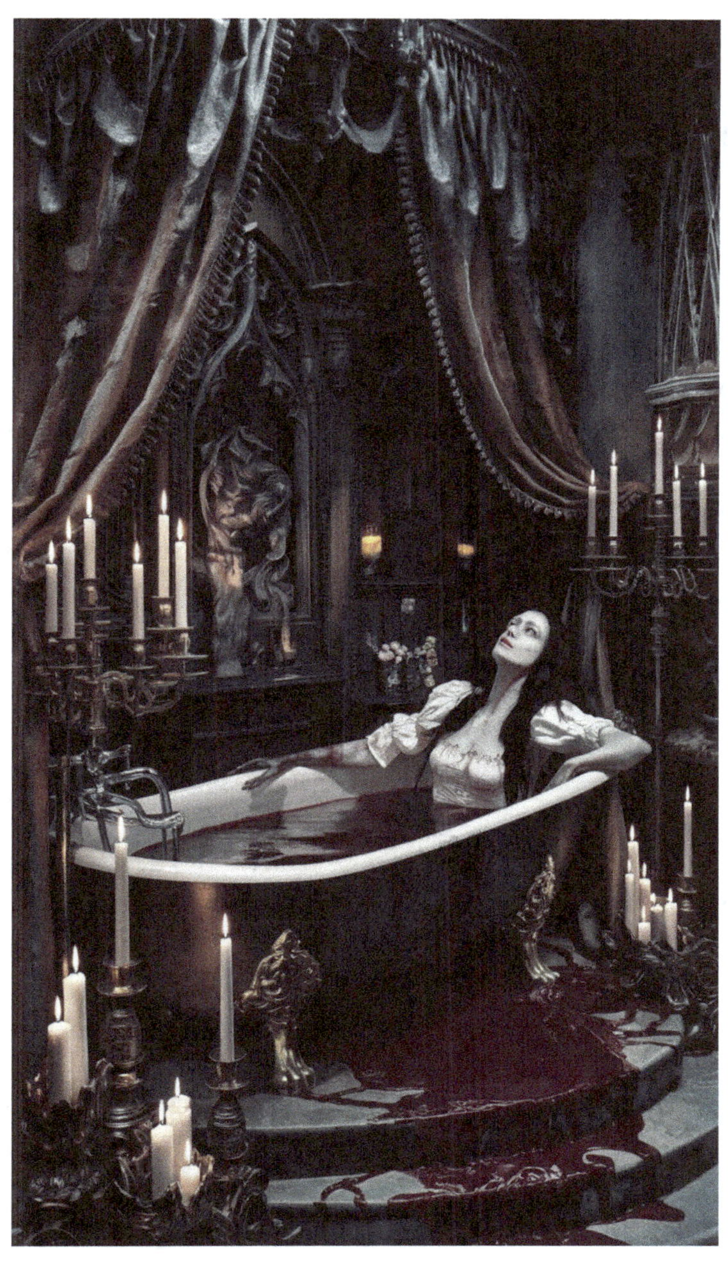

Elizabeth Bathory: The Blood Countess

In the lavish courts of Renaissance Europe, the pursuit of a flawless, porcelain complexion reached new levels of risk and indulgence. Noblewomen, draped in luxurious silks and sparkling jewels, turned to white lead-based cosmetics to mimic the fair skin of their admired goddesses. But beneath this elegant appearance was a hidden danger. The use of ceruse—a toxic mix of lead and vinegar—posed serious risks, leading to lead poisoning for those who applied it regularly. This pursuit of beauty came with a dangerous cost, leaving its mark on those who dared to flirt with such peril.

The Temptation of Faustian Bargains: A Dance with the Supernatural

The idea of striking a deal with the devil, known as a Faustian bargain, comes from the classic tale of Faust—a scholar whose hunger for knowledge pushes him to make a pact with the devil. Rooted in German folklore, Faust's story is a powerful warning about the dangers of trading one's soul for short-lived earthly pleasures. But Faust's tale is just one piece of a larger collection of folklore and myths that tell of people lured by the promise of eternal youth or unlimited power.

Stories of Faustian bargains appear across cultures and throughout history, echoing through myths and legends. In Jewish and Islamic traditions, the tale of King Solomon's deal with the demon Asmodeus highlights this timeless theme of trading one's soul for supernatural powers. Similarly, European folklore is full of stories about witches, sorcerers, and those practicing dark magic who make pacts with demons in exchange for wealth, power, or the secret to eternal youth.

Modern Echoes

Even today, the idea of Faustian bargains continues to fascinate audiences in many forms of media. Stephen Vincent Benet's eerie short story *"The Devil and Daniel Webster"* and the intense film *"The Devil's Advocate"* both explore the classic battle between temptation and morality. These modern takes remind us just how relevant Faustian stories remain in our shared culture. They show that the struggle between desires and values is as compelling now as it ever was.

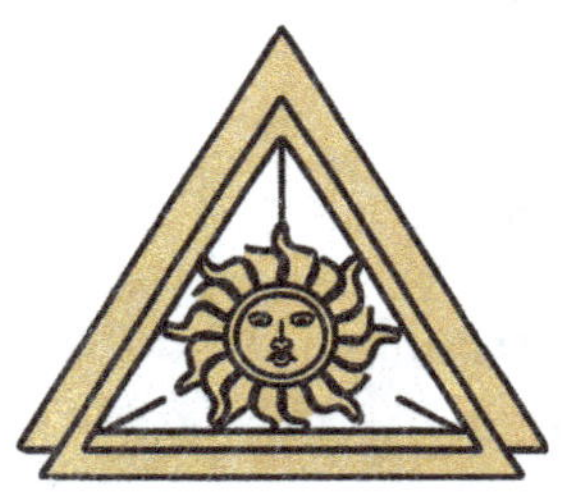

Chapter 4: Unveiling the Fountain of Youth

The mystery of the fountain of youth reflects humanity's refusal to accept that beauty lies in the seasons of life, not its permanence.

Throughout human history, few legends have captured as much attention and fascination as the tale of the Fountain of Youth—a mystical spring believed to have the incredible power to restore youth to those who drink from it. This intriguing story has appeared across cultures and throughout time, making its way into ancient texts, folklore, and myths. It symbolizes humanity's timeless desire to push back against aging and achieve immortality. The legend of the Fountain of Youth is a powerful reminder of our deep-rooted wish to defy time and hold onto youth forever.

The Mystic Waters

The Fountain of Youth has long been a symbol of humanity's unending quest for eternal youth and energy. Traces of this legendary spring can be found in Greek mythology, where tales of its rejuvenating powers have echoed through the centuries. Ancient texts from various cultures, including those from China, also mention an "Elixir of Life," a mystical substance believed to grant immortality to those who consume it.

The Age of Exploration

During the Age of Exploration, the legend of the Fountain of Youth gained even more attention, thanks to the stories told by bold explorers and adventurers. One of the most famous was the Spanish conquistador Juan Ponce de León, who set out on an expedition to the newly discovered Americas in the early 16th century. His goal? To find the legendary Fountain of Youth, which was rumored to be hidden somewhere in the lush, green landscapes of what is now Florida. Although his search ended without success, the tale of the Fountain of Youth continued to spark the imaginations of explorers and settlers, inspiring many more journeys in pursuit of eternal youth.

The Myth in Modernity

Over the centuries, the legend of the Fountain of Youth has gone beyond being just a myth or piece of folklore, making its way into art, literature, and pop culture. From medieval tapestries showing daring knights on their quest, to modern films and novels that dive into the timeless draw of immortality, the legend continues to fascinate audiences around the world. But more than just a fantasy story, the Fountain of Youth acts as a powerful symbol of humanity's deepest fears and dreams. It reflects our desire to go beyond the limits of mortality and find meaning in the face of eternity.

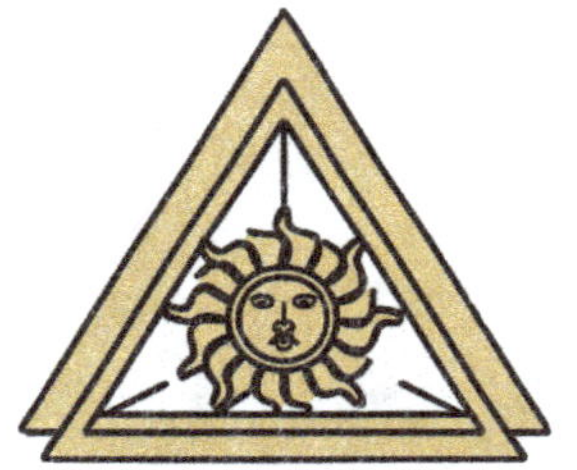

Chapter 5: Unraveling the Enigma of "Gold Juice"

The desire for immortality is not about living forever, but about the fear of being forgotten.

Whispers about a mysterious substance called "gold juice" have recently captured the attention of Hollywood and beyond, where fame and fortune are constantly sought after. The buzz began when actress Taryn Manning mentioned it during an interview on Whitney Cummings' podcast, *Good For You,* sparking widespread curiosity. Manning hinted at its connection to success and wealth but expressed caution, suggesting potential dangers tied to its allure. As the term "gold juice" spread across social media and became a trending topic on Google, people's imaginations went into overdrive. This enigmatic elixir, rumored to bestow fame and fortune on those daring enough to use it, has fascinated not only industry insiders but also everyday individuals eager to uncover its mystery. The idea plays into humanity's age-old fascination with the unknown, tapping into our endless curiosity about the secrets that might lie beneath the surface.

Taryn Manning's mention of "gold juice" sent waves through Hollywood's elite circles and quickly spread across the internet. Her cautious yet intriguing description left people curious and hungry for more details. Speculation took off, with theories ranging from the wildly imaginative to the eerily sinister. Some thought "gold juice" was a metaphor for the allure and temptation of fame and fortune in Hollywood, while others believed it might be an actual substance with strange, mysterious qualities. The buzz only added to the mystique, fueling discussions and questions about what it truly represents.

To understand why "gold juice" captivates so many, it's important to look at the mindset of those in the world of fame and celebrity. In an industry where image is everything and success often depends on perception, the idea of a secret elixir that could boost fame and fortune is undeniably tempting. For actors and actresses trying to carve out a name in an unforgiving field, the promise of a quick path to stardom is almost irresistible. The allure of something that could fast-track their rise to success speaks to the deep desire for recognition and the pressure to stand out.

Rumors and whispers have always surrounded the world of fame, revealing a hidden side full of secrets, scandals, and conspiracies. The recent mention of "gold juice" reignited longstanding beliefs about secret societies and powerful, unseen forces controlling the entertainment industry. Stories of celebrities trading their souls for fame and success have been shared for years, but the idea of an actual substance that could make such pacts possible adds a whole new layer. It takes these age-old tales to another level, stirring up even more curiosity and speculation.

As "gold juice" continued to trend online, driven by curiosity and wild speculation, people began to question if there was more to Taryn Manning's cryptic comments than they first thought. Was she hinting at something darker beneath Hollywood's polished surface? Or was it just a case of a celebrity using a metaphor, not realizing the buzz her words would create? The mystery kept everyone guessing and added even more intrigue to an already captivating story.

No matter what the truth behind Manning's comments really was, one thing was obvious: the idea of "gold juice" had captured the public's attention and sparked a worldwide conversation about fame and success in Hollywood. For many, it was a reminder of the powerful influence of celebrity and the timeless appeal of mystery and intrigue. As the buzz around "gold juice" started to settle, one question lingered: what secrets might still be hidden in the shadows of Hollywood's shining exterior?

Unveiling the Adrenochrome Myth

In the intricate space where science, literature, and the human mind meet, a mysterious compound called adrenochrome has captured the curiosity of both scholars and conspiracy theorists. Its origins are tied to the writings of influential figures like Aldous Huxley and Humphry Osmond, sparking fascination among those who explore the mysteries of consciousness and the human psyche. This compound has a way of drawing in those who are eager to dive deep into the unexplored corners of the mind.

Aldous Huxley and Humphry Osmond, pioneers in the fields of psychedelic research and literature, ventured into the unexplored world of altered states of consciousness. Their joint efforts in studying the effects of hallucinogens like mescaline and LSD earned them a significant place in both scientific and literary history. Their work opened doors to understanding the mind in new and fascinating ways, blending science with storytelling.

During their groundbreaking research, Huxley and Osmond came across an intriguing compound called adrenochrome—a metabolite of adrenaline found in the human body. Speculation soon swirled about its possible psychoactive effects, similar to those of other hallucinogens. This sparked a wave of fascination that captured the attention of researchers and the public alike, adding another layer of mystery to their studies.

It's important to separate speculation from solid evidence. Although Huxley and Osmond's conversations about adrenochrome suggested it might play a role in altered states of consciousness, the scientific community remained cautious. Researchers were waiting for concrete proof to back up these intriguing ideas before drawing any conclusions.

Even without solid scientific backing, the mention of adrenochrome in hallucinogenic research by respected figures like Huxley and Osmond pushed it into the realm of myth and intrigue. Its appeal went beyond the academic world, seeping into popular culture and fueling conspiracy theories where fact and fiction mix in an enticing blend of speculation and curiosity. This mystique kept people fascinated, drawing attention from both serious researchers and the public alike.

Over the years, mentions of adrenochrome have popped up in literature, movies, and even the darker corners of the internet, feeding its legend and linking it to stories of secret rituals and hidden societies. Yet, despite all the conspiracy theories swirling around, the true nature of adrenochrome remains uncertain. It's a captivating mystery that continues to draw in those curious enough to explore its depths.

Fear and Adrenochrome in Las Vegas

Hunter S. Thompson's *"Fear and Loathing in Las Vegas"* stands out as a defining piece of American literature, leaving an unforgettable mark on readers. The novel dives into chaotic, drug-infused adventures mixed with moments of existential introspection, where reality and hallucination intertwine. It follows a desperate search for meaning, drawing readers into a world where the pursuit of truth feels both urgent and unattainable.

At the heart of this intense story is the mysterious substance known as adrenochrome—a name that's spoken in whispers, cloaked in myth and intrigue. In the distorted, chaotic world of Thompson's protagonist, adrenochrome becomes the ultimate prize, a powerful elixir rumored to open the doors of perception and unlock new realms of experience.

As the protagonist navigates his drug-fueled journey through the neon-lit streets of Las Vegas, the search for adrenochrome becomes an all-consuming obsession, pushing him to the edge of madness and beyond. With each surreal and hallucinatory twist, Thompson brings adrenochrome to life as a mystical, elusive substance—temptingly just out of reach but impossible to resist.

Thompson's depiction of adrenochrome as a sought-after drug with powerful psychoactive effects resonated deeply with readers, capturing their imaginations and fueling intense speculation. Through the vivid and chaotic world of his writing, adrenochrome evolved from a simple byproduct of adrenaline into a symbol of existential angst and the pursuit of transcendence.

Amidst the chaos and wildness of *Fear and Loathing in Las Vegas,* there's a deeper truth—a reflection of the human experience and the constant search for meaning in a world that feels unhinged. Thompson's portrayal of adrenochrome acts as a metaphor for the quest for enlightenment in the face of existential despair. It's a journey into the depths of darkness where the line between reality and illusion blurs, leaving readers to question what's real and what's not.

As readers journey further into the twisted world of Thompson's story, they're pulled into a place where reality constantly shifts, and the line between sanity and madness starts to blur. In the intense haze of adrenochrome, they catch glimpses of both the darkest parts of human nature and moments of profound insight—a powerful mix of fear and revelation that stays with them long after they've finished the book.

The Myth and Mystique of Adrenochrome

Rumors about adrenochrome suggest that it's harvested from the adrenal glands of terrified individuals, fueling wild claims about its effects. Some believe it's a recreational drug favored by the elite, while others think it could be the secret to eternal youth and vitality. However, despite all the speculation and dramatic stories, one thing is clear: there is no scientific evidence to back up these claims.

The fascination with adrenochrome goes beyond its rumored effects; it taps into a deeper societal obsession with hidden powers and secret knowledge. In a world where trust in institutions and authority is waning, the idea of a mysterious substance capable of defying aging and mortality holds an undeniable allure. But it's this very allure that makes adrenochrome so captivating—and potentially dangerous—a symbol of our collective obsession with the unknown and the forbidden.

Separating Fact from Fiction on Gold Juice Plasma

The term "gold juice plasma" is another mysterious phrase that has captured people's imaginations. Conspiracy theorists have spun elaborate stories, claiming that a secret group of elites consumes blood taken from tortured children to obtain adrenochrome. However, a closer look shows a clear divide between these sensational claims and reality.

At the center of the "gold juice plasma" conspiracy is a tangled web of misinformation and sensationalism. The idea that elites consume blood plasma from tortured children to achieve youth and vitality is both shocking and fantastical. Yet, despite the absence of credible evidence to support such claims, these stories continue to thrive in the darker corners of the internet and popular culture.

While there is legitimate research into the potential benefits of plasma transfusions, especially from young donors, the idea that these practices can reverse aging remains speculative and unproven. The scientific community stresses the importance of evidence-based research and encourages critical thinking when assessing such claims. For most people, the concept of using blood plasma infusions to rejuvenate the body and turn back the clock on aging feels far-fetched and beyond the bounds of reality

The ethical issues surrounding the idea of harvesting blood from unwilling or exploited individuals for adrenochrome or other supposed benefits are extremely concerning. The exploitation and abuse of vulnerable people in the pursuit of youth and longevity raise serious moral questions that can't be ignored. Any claims about using "gold juice plasma" should be approached with skepticism and careful examination, not only from a scientific perspective but also from an ethical standpoint.

Chapter 6: Liquid Gold Therapy Beyond the Conspiracy

A life filled with beauty begins with the decision to see it everywhere: in nature, in others, and most importantly, in yourself.

In contrast to the many conspiracy theories out there, liquid gold therapy is a genuine medical practice. Known as platelet-rich plasma (PRP) therapy, this technique uses the body's own healing properties to stimulate tissue repair and regeneration. It involves taking a patient's blood, isolating the platelets with growth factors, and re-injecting them into targeted areas. This approach shows promising applications in both medicine and cosmetic dermatology.

Platelet-rich plasma (PRP) therapy has its roots in the 1970s, when researchers first started studying the regenerative properties of platelets. Over the years, advancements in medical technology have transformed PRP therapy into a safe and effective treatment option. Today, it's used for a variety of conditions, including orthopedic injuries, wound healing, and hair loss.

Leading the way in PRP research is Dr. Robert A. Marx, whose groundbreaking studies in the 1990s helped establish PRP therapy as a viable medical treatment. Through careful research, Dr. Marx demonstrated PRP's effectiveness in promoting healing in bone and soft tissue across various fields, including orthopedics, dental work, and plastic surgery. His clinical trials showed that PRP could enhance bone growth, support tissue repair, and reduce complications after surgery, setting a strong foundation for its use in medical treatments.

In cosmetic dermatology, liquid gold therapy, or PRP therapy, has become a popular non-invasive option for skin rejuvenation. By boosting collagen production and encouraging tissue repair, PRP therapy can enhance skin texture, tone, and elasticity. It has shown promising results in treating acne scars, fine lines, wrinkles, and uneven pigmentation, offering a natural approach to achieving a fresher, more youthful appearance.

While PRP therapy's effectiveness for different conditions is still being studied, its potential as a non-invasive treatment for rejuvenation is clear. Clinical studies have shown that PRP can help speed up wound healing, reduce inflammation, and support tissue regeneration. However, further research is needed to fully understand how it works and to refine treatment protocols for the best results.

Despite its promising benefits, liquid gold therapy does come with some limitations and risks. Like any medical procedure, PRP therapy can lead to side effects such as pain, swelling, bruising, and even infection.

Additionally, its efficacy can vary depending on factors such as the patient's age, overall health, and the specific condition being treated.

The rise of liquid gold therapy shows the importance of teamwork among researchers, clinicians, and industry professionals in advancing medical science. By blending innovative technology with careful scientific study, we can tap into the full potential of PRP therapy and bring transformative changes to regenerative medicine.

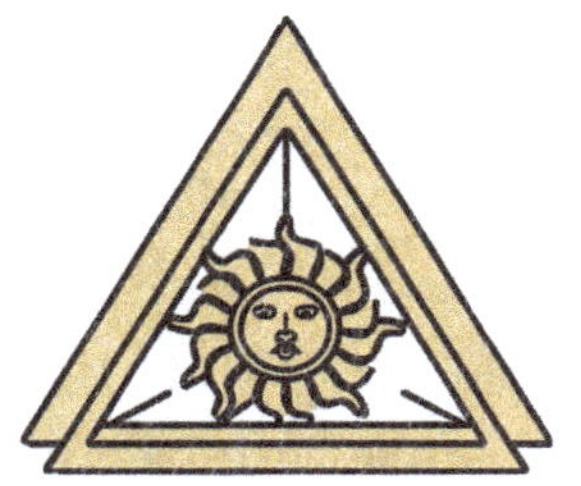

Chapter 7: Youthful Blood Transfusions

The greatest injustice is a legacy where the young inherit the debris of selfishness while the old live without accountability.

If you're a millennial, you might have felt for a while that older generations seem to be draining us dry. Many millennials feel a sense of resentment, seeing previous generations as having enjoyed more stable economic conditions, while younger people today grapple with things like student loan debt and sky-high housing prices. This sense of imbalance can lead to feelings of being exploited or "sucked dry" by older generations who haven't fully addressed these systemic issues. And lately, this idea of "bloodsucking" seems to have taken on a more literal twist.

Enter the controversial trend of wealthy individuals infusing themselves with the blood of young people in hopes of slowing down the aging process. This unusual approach, based on the idea that youthful blood might hold the secret to rejuvenation, has sparked a mix of fascination, debate, and ethical concerns.

More than 100 people have taken part in a clinical trial at a San Francisco startup in 2016 that offers blood transfusions specifically for older adults. Each session, costing a hefty $8,000 (£6,200), involves transfusing two and a half liters of plasma—the liquid part of blood—sourced from young donors. The median age of participants in this experimental treatment is around 60.

Liquid Gold: Exploring the Mysteries of Plasma

In the complex makeup of blood, plasma stands out for its unique qualities and essential functions. Often called "liquid gold" for its golden-yellow color, plasma makes up about 55% of our blood's volume. Its color isn't just for show; it reflects the rich mix of proteins and lipids that make this fluid so vital to our bodies.

Plasma plays a vital role in transporting essential components throughout the body. It carries oxygen-rich red blood cells, infection-fighting white blood cells, clot-forming platelets, and important nutrients and electrolytes. Acting as the lifeline of the circulatory system, plasma helps exchange substances between tissues, regulates osmotic pressure, and maintains the delicate balance needed for our bodies to function smoothly.

Plasma's golden color comes from the proteins and lipids that make up its composition. Albumin, one of the most abundant proteins in plasma, plays a major role in giving plasma its color. Additionally, lipids like cholesterol and triglycerides contribute to the golden hue by scattering and absorbing certain wavelengths of light as it passes through plasma.

Beyond its color, plasma plays a crucial role in supporting the body's immune system. Packed with antibodies and immune cells, plasma serves as a frontline defense against pathogens and infections, strengthening the body's ability to resist disease and stay resilient.

In regenerative medicine, plasma stands out as a symbol of hope, showcasing the body's natural ability to heal and renew. Its golden color is a reminder of the preciousness of life, capturing the vitality and resilience that flows through our veins.

Revolutionizing Anti-Aging: The Promise of Young Blood Plasma

In the field of anti-aging research, Jesse Karmazin is a notable figure pushing the boundaries of rejuvenation therapy. With a Stanford background and a drive for biomedical innovation, Karmazin founded a U.S. clinic to explore a unique approach: transfusing young blood plasma from donors into older recipients. His method has sparked both interest and controversy.

Karmazin's clinic, Ambrosia, has generated significant excitement, with early patient trials showing promising results in 2016. The potential benefits are impressive—not only does Karmazin suggest improvements in appearance, but he also highlights a range of health benefits, from better diabetes management to enhanced cognitive function. These bold claims suggest a groundbreaking treatment that could reshape the future of anti-aging therapies.

As with any pioneering approach, Karmazin's work has been met with some skepticism. Concerns around the rigor of clinical evidence and ethical questions raise the need for caution and further study. Critics emphasize the importance of thorough research and regulatory oversight to confirm the safety and effectiveness of young blood plasma transfusions for anti-aging.

In response to growing scrutiny, Karmazin firmly defends his study, stating that it has passed thorough ethical reviews and arguing that giving placebos to paying participants would be unfair. He highlights the real benefits patients have reported so far, describing the treatment as "plastic surgery from the inside out." This bold comparison suggests a level of rejuvenation that goes beyond surface improvements, hinting at deeper cellular or physiological renewal.

Despite the challenges, Karmazin's efforts represent a bold step into new territory. His vision and dedication highlight the drive for innovation in the quest to slow the aging process. As anti-aging science advances, young blood plasma therapy remains an intriguing area, inspiring both hope and skepticism in equal parts

The idea of using young blood to rejuvenate older individuals isn't entirely new. Over the past 17 years, multiple studies, including those at Stanford University, have shown promising effects in mice. These studies have found that when the circulatory systems of old and young mice are connected—a process called parabiosis—organs, muscles, and stem cells in the older mice show signs of rejuvenation. More recent findings also suggest that injecting young plasma into older mice has similar rejuvenating effects.

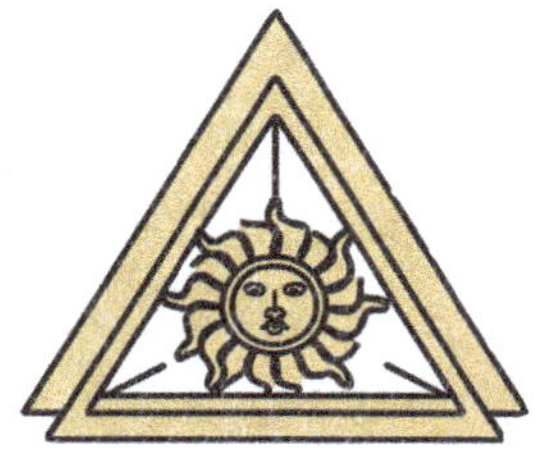

Chapter 8: The Eternal Quest for Youth

Mortality is both our greatest fear and our greatest gift, urging us to cherish each fleeting breath.

The human obsession with staying young reflects some of our deepest fears and desires. Within us is a natural drive to find ways to slow down or reverse aging, even as we're inevitably moving closer to the reality of mortality. This desire to preserve youth touches on fundamental aspects of the human experience, showing how powerful our instincts are when it comes to facing the passage of time.

Fear of Mortality

Aging, with its unmistakable effects on our bodies and minds, is a powerful reminder of our mortality, confronting us with life's finite nature. As beings with self-awareness, we carry an understanding of our own mortality throughout life. Every wrinkle, gray hair, and slight decline in physical ability is a visible sign of time passing, bringing us closer to life's inevitable end.

The deep-rooted fear of mortality is a powerful force in human consciousness, pushing many to seek ways to hold onto youth and vitality. Faced with life's inevitable end, we naturally cling to life, wanting to keep our physical and mental abilities intact as long as possible. This fear of aging motivates us to try everything from lifestyle adjustments to medical treatments in hopes of slowing down the passage of time.

The fear of mortality ultimately drives personal growth, encouraging us to reflect on life's fleeting nature and the importance of making the most of our time. While aging is unavoidable, how we respond to it —whether through acceptance, resilience, or taking proactive steps—shapes our journey toward a fulfilling, meaningful life, even with the awareness of life's limits.

Cultural Ideals and Societal Pressure

Cultural ideals and social pressures strongly shape how we view youth and beauty, influencing both our self-image and our perceptions of others as we age. In many cultures, youthfulness is linked to qualities like desirability, success, and vitality, creating an ideal that people often strive to reach and hold onto throughout their lives.

From an early age, people are flooded with messages that celebrate youth and, at the same time, cast aging in a negative light. These messages show up everywhere— in flawless celebrity images in the media and ads for anti-aging products and procedures. This constant exposure creates a strong pressure to keep a youthful look, leading many to internalize unrealistic beauty standards and feel self-conscious as they grow older.

This pressure is especially intense for women, who often face more scrutiny and judgment based on their looks. They're constantly receiving messages that stress how youthfulness is key to attracting partners, moving forward in their careers, and keeping social status. As a result, many women feel pushed to spend significant time, energy, and money trying to stay youthful—sometimes at the cost of their own physical and emotional well-being.

The pressure to look youthful can feel overwhelming, often pushing people toward extreme measures to resist aging and meet unrealistic beauty standards. From invasive cosmetic procedures to strict dieting and intense workout routines, this pursuit can impact both physical and mental health, leading to body dissatisfaction, low self-esteem, and even disordered eating habits.

The cultural focus on youthfulness can also fuel ageism—a bias against people based on their age. Older individuals may feel marginalized and overlooked in many areas of life, from the workplace and healthcare to media representation. This pressure to hide signs of aging and maintain a youthful look only adds to the challenges they face.

Cultural standards and societal pressure have a huge impact on how we see aging and beauty. These ideals often shape how people think and act, creating a tricky balance between what we truly want and what we feel like we're supposed to want. But here's the good news: we can question these deeply rooted beliefs. By doing that, we open the door to a world where everyone—no matter their age—is valued and celebrated. It's about creating a space that respects individuality, highlights the beauty in diversity, and embraces aging as something natural and meaningful.

Biological Instincts

Our biological instincts have a lot to do with how we feel about aging and the constant quest to look and feel young. From an evolutionary angle, staying youthful and healthy has always been tied to survival and reproduction—it's just built into us. Historically, youth has been seen as a sign of fertility and vitality, which made it a highly sought-after trait when it came to choosing a mate and ensuring the continuation of our species. This natural connection to reproductive success explains why society often places such a high value on looking and feeling young.

The natural urge to hold onto youthfulness comes from an evolutionary need to keep the next generation thriving. Back in the day, life was tough—harsh environments and high death rates meant survival wasn't guaranteed. People who showed signs of youth and vitality were more likely to attract partners and have children, passing their genes along to the next generation. Over time, this led to natural selection favoring traits and behaviors linked to staying youthful and fit for reproduction. This cycle helped ensure the survival of the species, keeping life moving forward.

The deep-rooted desire to stay youthful is still a major influence on how people think and act today, even though it shows up in more complex and subtle ways. Thanks to advancements in medicine and technology, we're living longer and have better tools to deal with the challenges of aging. But despite these improvements, the natural drive to look and feel young hasn't gone away—it's still very much a part of how we're wired. It's like a whisper in the back of our minds, reminding us of our instinctive connection to health, vitality, and survival.

In today's world, youthfulness is often linked to beauty, energy, and even social status, which adds to the pressure to maintain a youthful look. For many, the instinct to hold onto their youth goes beyond just appearance—it's about boosting their chances in love, advancing in their careers, and even living longer. This drive to fight the aging process shows up in all kinds of ways. People might adopt healthier habits, invest in anti-aging skincare routines, or turn to medical treatments designed to help them look and feel younger. It's a modern take on an age-old desire to stay vibrant and full of life.

The fear of aging and the awareness of our own mortality, both deeply tied to our biological instincts, often push people to explore anti-aging treatments and solutions. It's not just about wrinkles or gray hair—it's about resisting the decline that comes with getting older. This deep-seated drive to stay youthful has been with humanity for centuries, influencing behaviors and fueling the ongoing search for ways to extend life and maintain vitality. Whether through skincare, advanced medical procedures, or lifestyle changes, this pursuit reflects our instinctive desire to hold onto our energy and zest for as long as possible.

Biological instincts play a powerful role in shaping how we think and act when it comes to aging and chasing youthfulness. These natural drives, combined with cultural and societal influences, create a complex mix that shapes our views on age and beauty. Understanding how these instincts work is key to making sense of human behavior and tackling the many challenges that come with aging in today's world. By recognizing these deep-rooted influences, we can start to approach aging with more awareness and empathy, paving the way for a healthier, more balanced perspective.

Psychological Factors

Aging isn't just about physical changes—it's a complex process that also brings significant psychological and emotional shifts. These changes play a big role in shaping how people see themselves and their sense of identity. As they get older, individuals often face a range of challenges and transitions that can affect their mental well-being and overall quality of life. From adapting to new roles to processing life's milestones, the journey of aging touches every part of who we are.

One of the biggest mental and emotional challenges of aging is dealing with the loss of youthfulness and the changes that come with it—like shifts in physical appearance, health, and even cognitive abilities. For many, getting older can feel like a dramatic change from their younger selves, with wrinkles, gray hair, and less physical energy serving as constant reminders. These visible signs of aging can bring up feelings of insecurity, self-doubt, and vulnerability, especially when they're tied to a sense of losing attractiveness, vitality, or social standing. It's a tough transition that affects not just how people see themselves but also how they think the world sees them.

Aging often comes with changes in health and cognitive abilities, which can add another layer of emotional and mental challenges. As people notice their physical health or mental sharpness declining, it can feel like they're losing their sense of independence and control. Simple things like mobility, memory, or the ability to handle daily tasks might start to slip, leading to feelings of frustration, helplessness, and even fear about relying on others for support. These shifts can be overwhelming, making it harder to maintain a sense of autonomy and confidence as they navigate this stage of life.

The process of aging often brings significant changes in social roles, relationships, and expectations, which can have a profound effect on a person's sense of identity and self-worth. As individuals age, they may find their social networks shifting—through the loss of loved ones, stepping away from the workforce, or taking on new caregiving responsibilities. These transitions can upend familiar routines, weaken social bonds, and challenge the sources of meaning and fulfillment they once relied on. This can lead to feelings of loneliness, isolation, and a deep sense of questioning about life's purpose.

The psychological effects of aging are both complex and deeply personal, touching on a wide range of emotions, experiences, and challenges that shape how individuals see themselves and their overall well-being. By understanding and addressing these mental and emotional aspects, society can play a key role in improving the mental health and quality of life for older adults. Creating a more inclusive, supportive, and age-friendly environment not only benefits older generations but also helps foster respect and understanding across all age groups.

Aging is a natural part of life, but let's be real—it's not always easy to embrace. Society loves to put youth on a pedestal, acting like it's the only thing that matters. But here's the thing: getting older isn't something to fear or fight against. It's an experience we all share, a reminder that we're human and connected. Sure, the world might bombard us with anti-aging ads and endless messages about staying forever young, but the reality is that aging is a normal, beautiful process. It's also a chance to rethink how we live, challenge those outdated societal ideas, and discover new ways to find purpose and joy in every stage of life.

One of the most eye-opening truths about aging is realizing how universal it is. No matter who you are—rich or poor, famous or unknown, from any corner of the world—aging is something everyone goes through. It's a shared experience that levels the playing field, reminding us that we're all connected in this journey of life. When we embrace this reality, it opens the door to something powerful: empathy. Knowing that we're all facing the same ticking clock helps us feel more compassion for one another, creating a sense of solidarity that bridges gaps between generations and backgrounds. It's a humbling reminder of our shared humanity and how much we really have in common.

Embracing aging isn't just about accepting wrinkles or gray hairs—it's about recognizing the beauty and wisdom that come with getting older. Think about it: as people age, they gather a lifetime of stories, lessons, and insights that can make life richer not only for themselves but for everyone they interact with. Instead of seeing aging as some kind of loss or decline, it's better to reframe it as a time to appreciate how much you've learned and how far you've come. This shift in perspective can bring a deeper sense of self-acceptance, confidence, and even fulfillment. After all, there's something undeniably powerful about owning your experiences and using them to inspire others.

Finding meaning and purpose at every stage of life is a huge part of embracing the reality of aging. Instead of getting stuck wishing for the past or stressing about what's ahead, it's all about focusing on the here and now. Gratitude and mindfulness can be game-changers, helping people stay present and enjoy the moment. Building strong relationships, diving into activities that bring joy, and continuing to grow on a personal level are all ways to create a life that feels fulfilling no matter your age. Purpose isn't something that fades with time—it evolves, giving each chapter of life its own unique meaning.

Conclusion: The Hidden Layers of Conspiracy Culture

Mortality is not a curse but a reminder to love deeply, live fully, and leave a legacy that outlasts the body.

As we wrap up our journey through the fascinating world of *Gold Juice*, we've arrived at a crossroads full of intrigue and unanswered questions. Along the way, we've dived headfirst into the depths of conspiracy theories, sifting through layers of speculation and suspicion to uncover hidden truths. Now, as we step away from these mysterious waters, it's the perfect time to reflect on what we've uncovered and what still remains shrouded in mystery. While some pieces of the puzzle have fallen into place, others continue to tease us, leaving just enough to keep the curiosity alive.

Throughout history, conspiracy theories have always had a way of grabbing our attention, pulling us in with the promise of uncovering hidden truths and secret knowledge. But as we've explored, these theories are rarely straightforward. Behind each one lies a complicated mix of facts, wild speculation, and fictional twists—a blend that makes it hard to tell where reality ends and myth begins. It's this blurred line between what's real and what's imagined that keeps us hooked, always questioning and searching for answers.

Amid all the chaos and confusion, there are those rare moments when everything becomes clear—when the curtain is pulled back, and the truth is impossible to ignore. Think about the Watergate scandal. What started as whispers of conspiracy ended up shaking the core of American democracy, exposing a shocking level of political corruption. Or take Edward Snowden, whose brave decision to blow the whistle on the NSA's mass surveillance program confirmed what many had long suspected—that the government was overstepping its bounds and prying into private lives. These moments remind us that sometimes, conspiracy theories aren't just theories—they're uncomfortable truths waiting to be uncovered.

These examples are powerful reminders that conspiracy theories, while often brushed off as wild ideas from overly paranoid minds, can sometimes uncover pieces of truth that deserve a closer look. As we wade through the tricky waters of conspiracy culture, it's important to stay sharp. Separating fact from fiction takes effort, but it's worth it. By questioning the narratives we're given and staying open to critical thinking, we can approach these stories with both curiosity and caution, ensuring we don't overlook truths hidden in plain sight.

With *Gold Juice,* the allure of the unknown has pulled us deep into a world of speculation and endless theories. It's been a wild ride, unraveling clues and piecing together fragments of a mystery that seems just out of reach. But as we prepare to step away from this captivating puzzle, one thing remains certain: the truth has a way of coming to light, even if it takes time. Who knows? Maybe one day, the veil will be lifted, and the secrets of *Gold Juice* will finally be revealed, giving us the answers we've been chasing all along.

Until then, let's keep exploring, questioning, and digging beneath the surface to uncover the truths hidden in our world. The search for knowledge and understanding is a journey that can lead to some surprising discoveries. Who knows? Along the way, we might even expose the biggest conspiracy of all—the conspiracy of silence. It's the quiet force that works to keep us unaware and disconnected from the realities that shape our lives. By staying curious and refusing to settle for half-truths, we can challenge that silence and shine a light on the things that really matter.

As we say goodbye to *Gold Juice* and the mysteries it has brought to light, let's take a moment to hold on to the lessons we've learned and the truths we've uncovered. In the end, it's our curiosity, our healthy skepticism, and our determination to seek out the truth that will guide us. These are the tools that help us move beyond the shadows of doubt and into the clarity of understanding. The journey doesn't end here—it's just

another step forward into the pursuit of what lies
beneath the surface.

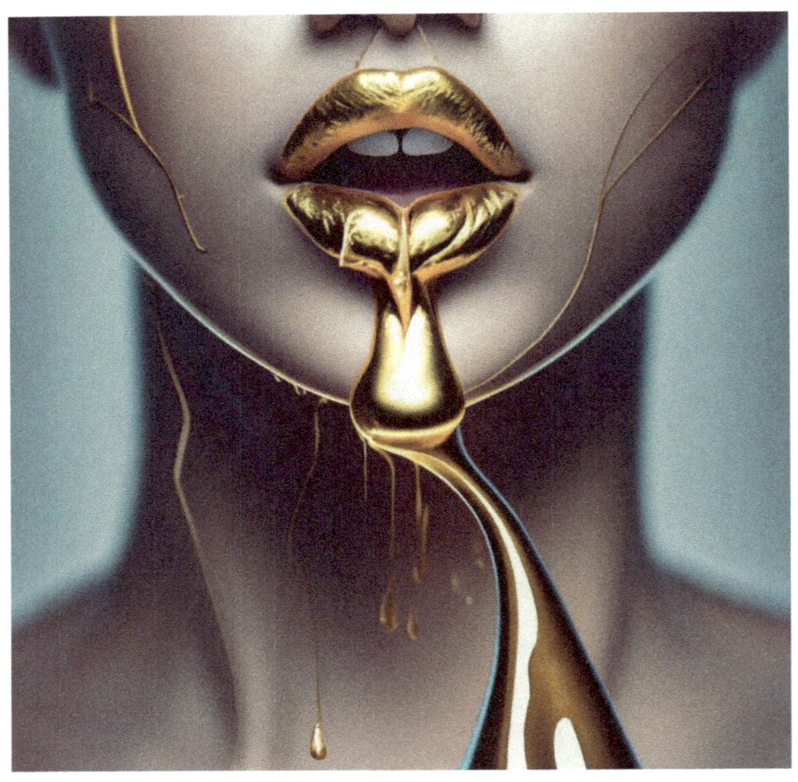

Liquid Gold: The Taste of Eternity

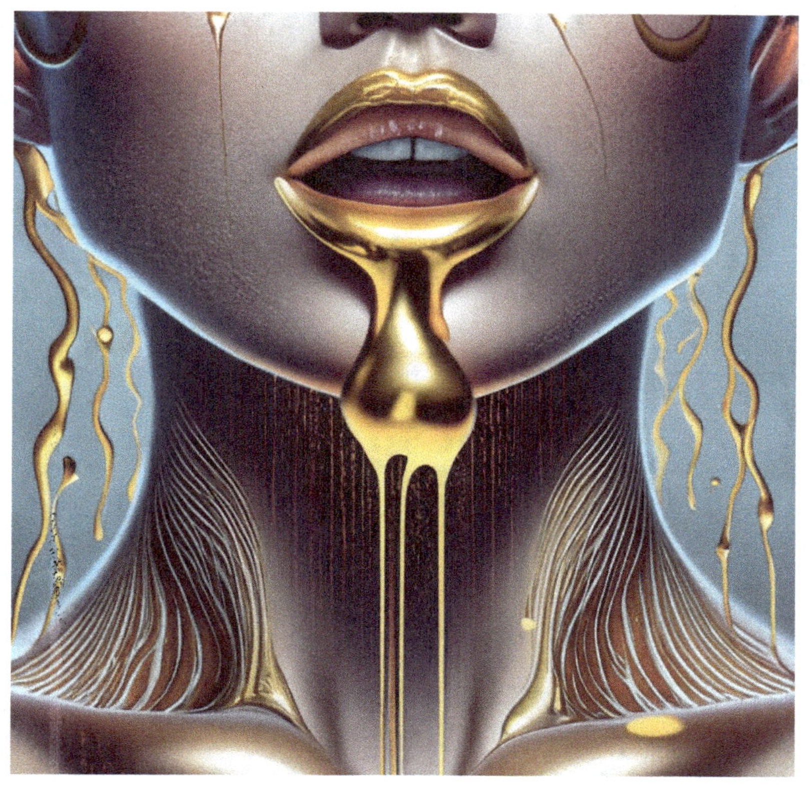

Gold Juice Lips of Lust

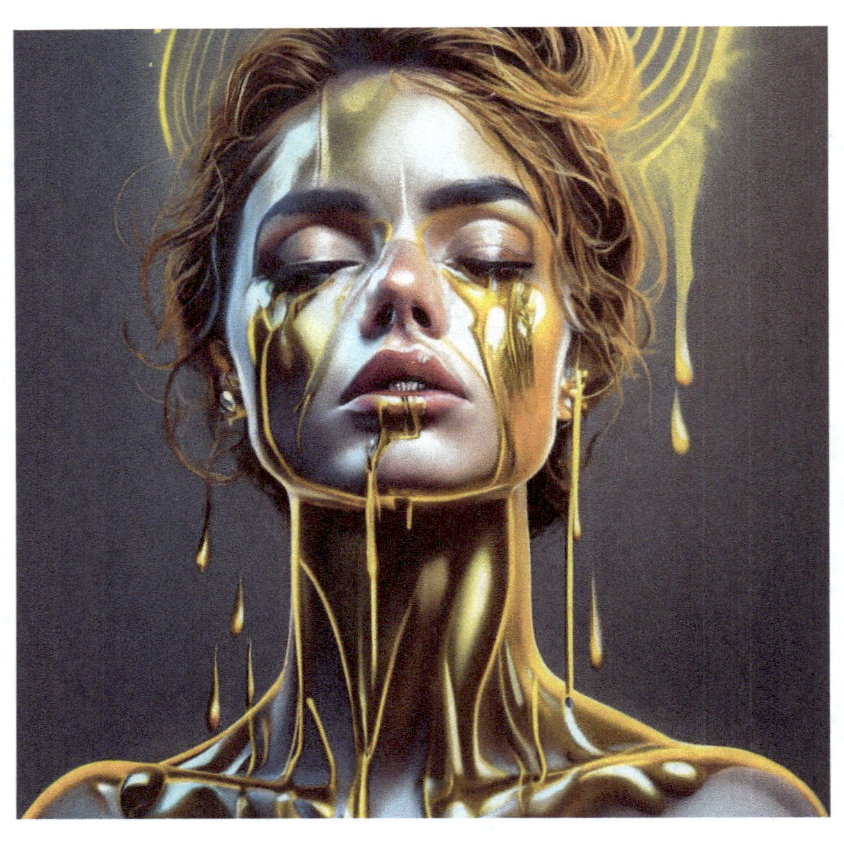

Gold Juice Veins of Eternity

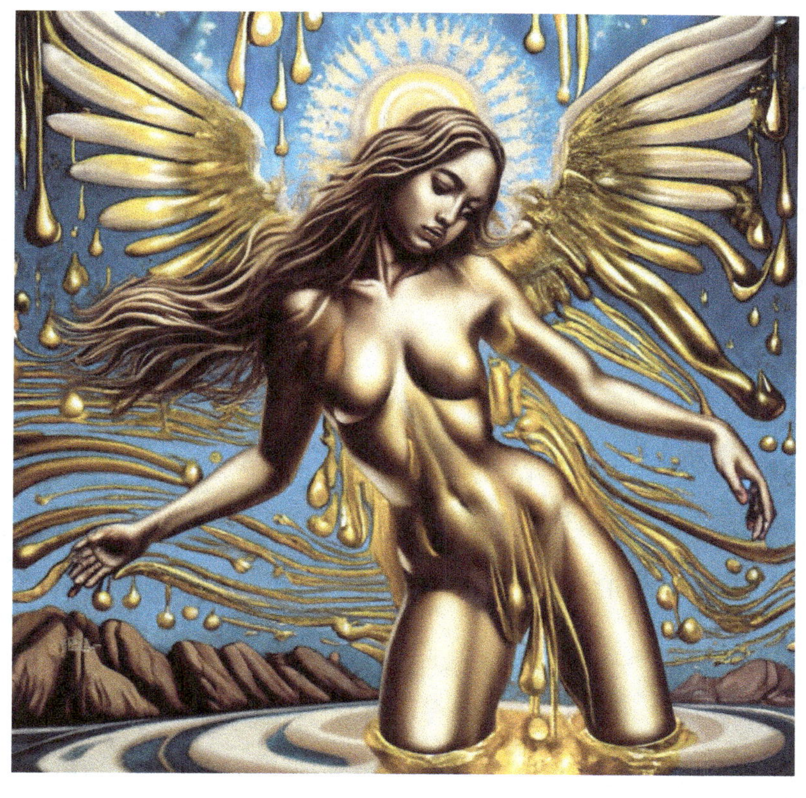

Gold Juice: The Divine Elixir

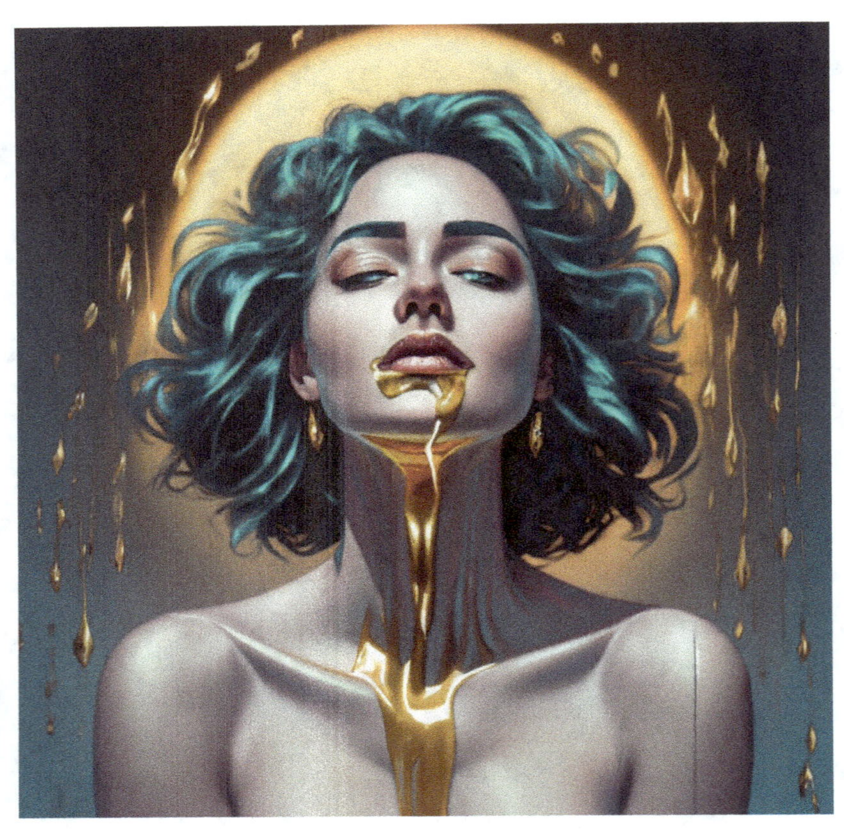

Gold Juice Cravings

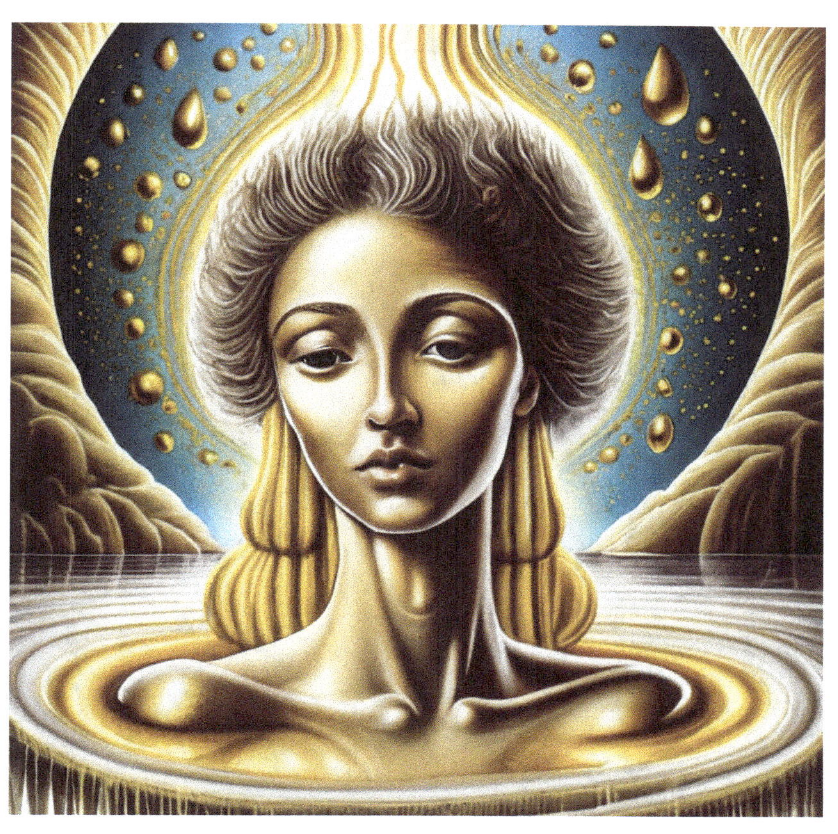

Gold Juice of Eternity

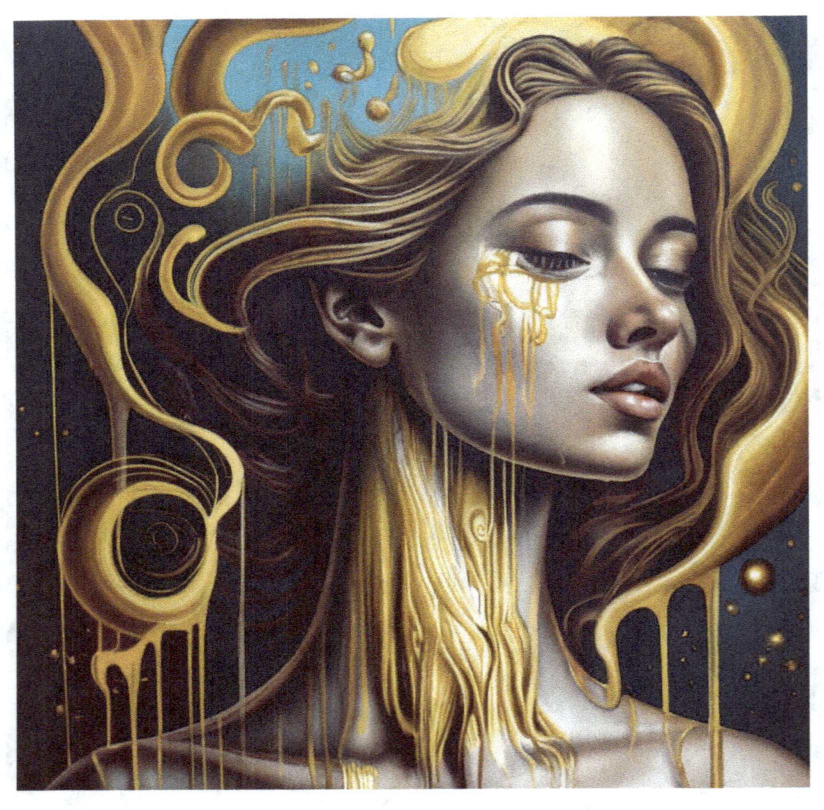

Gold Juice: Nectar of the Heavens

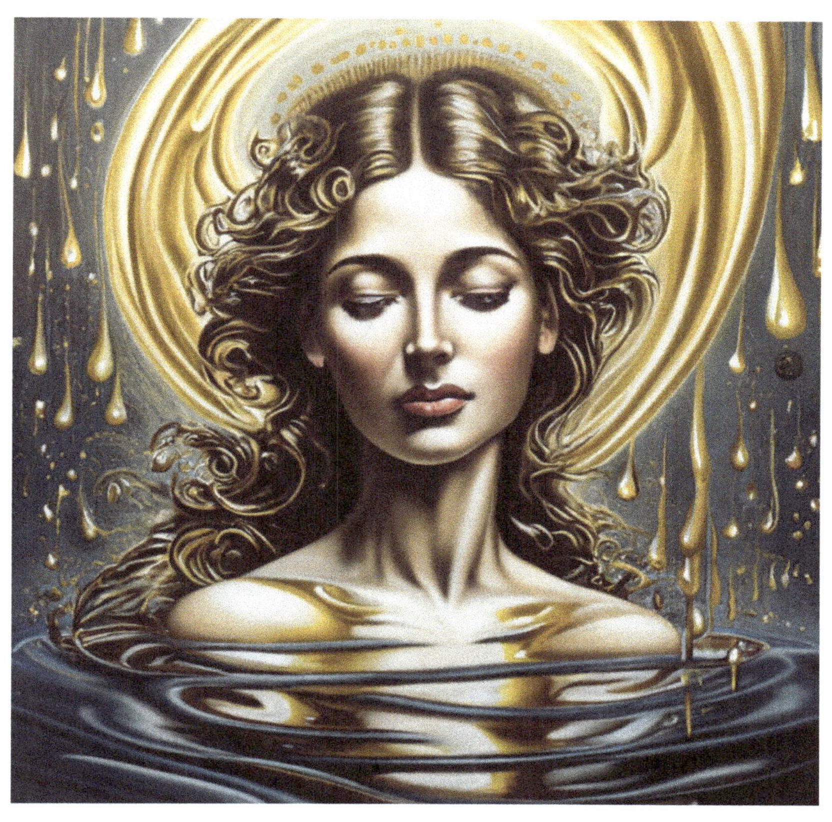

Gold Juice Drops of Divine

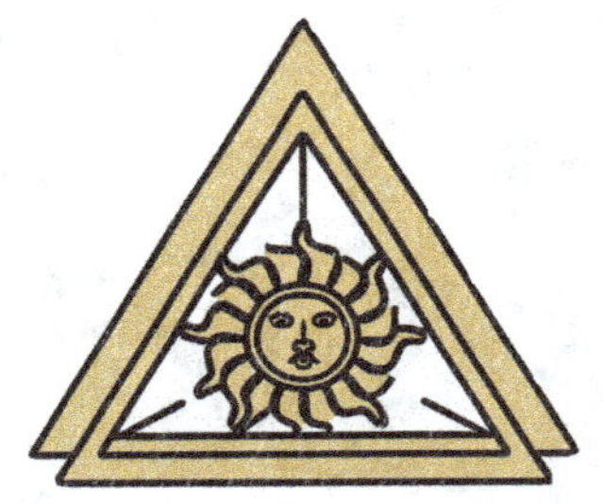